Comments on *Kidney Failure Explained* from readers

'*Kidney Failure Explained* remains the most sought after reference for kidney patients. Since the first edition appeared in 1999 the National Kidney Federation has continued to recommend this book above all others. As the treatment for kidney disease advances, so this book has kept pace. We wish the third edition well.'
Timothy F Statham OBE, Chief Executive,
National Kidney Federation

'I was so impressed by the wonderful way the book is presented, in terms which everyone can understand. Our committee has recommended the book to our members.'
Roy Bradbury, Chairman, Sheffield Area Kidney Association

'This is a very well written book and it should be of great value to renal patients.'
Professor R. Wilkinson, Consultant Nephrologist,
Freeman Group of Hospitals, Newcastle-upon-Tyne

'The book is excellent and will prove very valuable to a variety of different groups. I shall certainly be recommending it to patients and to general practitioners in particular.'
Dr Robin Winney, Consultant Renal Physician, Department of Renal Medicine, The Royal Infirmary of Edinburgh

'The content of the book is realistic but positive and covered all aspects of kidney failure. I have already started recommending it to some of my patients.'
Ros Tibbles, Pre-dialysis Sister, Department of Renal Medicine and Transplantation, The Royal Hospitals NHS Trust

Comments on *Kidney Failure Explained* (continued)

'This book is, without doubt, the best resource currently available
for kidney patients and those who care for them.'
Val Said, Kidney transplant patient

'*Kidney Failure Explained* not only answered all the questions
I wanted to ask, it also answered a lot of questions I hadn't even
thought of. Books of this kind are badly needed. Thank you
for a clear and precise text, in language I can understand.'
Dennis Jackson, CAPD patient

'Your book has been a tremendous help and support throughout.
I think that *Kidney Failure Explained* should be offered
to all renal patients.'
J. R., Kidney donor, Northampton

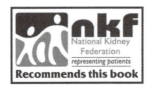

*The National Kidney Federation (NKF) is a charity representing all
kidney patients in the United Kingdom, it is run by Kidney patients
for Kidney patients. The Federation campaigns for increased renal
provision and improved treatment. The charity also provides
national services to assist all kidney patients.*

*Publications recommended by the NKF have to be of a high standard
and easily readable, the recommendation is not given lightly
and is highly prized. The NKF recommendation of this book
was made at the time of its publication and has to be renewed
at subsequent prints in order to retain the NKF endorsement and
recommendation. Further information about the NKF and books
it recommends can be found on its website www.kidney.org.uk.*

KIDNEY FAILURE EXPLAINED

Everything you always wanted to know about
dialysis and kidney transplants
but were afraid to ask

Dr Andy Stein, MD, FRCP

Consultant Nephrologist and Acute Physician, University Hospitals,
Coventry and Warwickshire NHS Trust

Janet Wild, RGN

Clinical Education Manager, Baxter Healthcare Ltd, Newbury, Berkshire

CLASS PUBLISHING • LONDON

Printing history
First published 1999
Printed with revisions 2000
Second edition 2002
Third edition 2007

10 9 8 7 6 5 4 3 2 1

The authors and publishers welcome feedback from the users of this book. Please contact the publishers.

Class Publishing, Barb House, Barb Mews, London W6 7PA, UK
Telephone: 020 7371 2119
Fax: 020 7371 2878 [International +4420]
email: post@class.co.uk
www.class.co.uk

The information presented in this book is accurate and current to the best of the authors' knowledge. The authors and publisher, however, make no guarantee as to, and assume no responsibility for, the correctness, sufficiency or completeness of such information or recommendation. The reader is advised to consult a doctor regarding all aspects of individual health care.

A CIP catalogue record for this book is available from the British Library

ISBN 10 1859591450
ISBN 13 9781859591451

Designed and illustrated by Darren Bennett

Edited by Richenda Milton-Thompson

Printed and bound in Slovenia by Delo Tiskarna
by arrangement with Presernova druzba

CONTENTS

FOREWORD TO THIS EDITION
Professor John Feehally   xi

ACKNOWLEDGEMENTS   xii

INTRODUCTION   xiii

1 WHAT IS KIDNEY FAILURE?
Introduction   1
Kidneys – what and where are they?   1
The kidneys' main job: making urine   1
Why make urine?   2
Removing toxic wastes   2
Removing excess water   3
Other functions of the kidneys   4
Kidney failure – what is it?   4
What are the symptoms?   5
How is kidney failure diagnosed?   5
What causes kidneys to fail?   5
The 'progression' of kidney failure   7
What is ERF?   7
How is ERF treated?   7
When should dialysis be started?   9
Can the need for dialysis be delayed?   9
Will dialysis or a transplant solve the problem?   10
Why treat kidney failure?   10
Key Facts   11

2 TOXIN 'CLEARANCE'
Introduction   12
Why is clearance measured?   12
How is clearance measured?   12
Why measure urea or creatinine?   13

Types of test   13
Blood tests for urea or creatinine   14
Blood creatinine before dialysis   14
Starting dialysis   14
Blood creatinine during dialysis   15
Blood creatinine with a transplant   15
Urea or creatinine clearance tests   16
How is clearance measured?   16
Urea or creatinine clearance during dialysis   17
The eGFR   17
So, is 'more dialysis' better?   18
Key Facts   18

3 FLUID BALANCE
Introduction   19
Flesh and fluid   19
What is the 'target weight'?   20
Control of fluid balance   20
Sodium and fluid balance   20
What is fluid overload?   21
How is fluid overload treated?   21
Dehydration   21
How is dehydration treated?   22
Taking control of your own fluid balance   22
Key Facts   23

4 BLOOD PRESSURE
Introduction   24
High blood pressure and kidney failure   24
Low blood pressure and kidney failure   24
Circulation of the blood   24
Measuring blood pressure   25
What is 'normal' blood pressure?   26

Does anxiety affect blood pressure? 26
How do you know that your blood pressure is high
  or low? 26
Why treat high blood pressure? 27
What determines blood pressure levels? 27
How is high blood pressure treated? 27
Are the blood pressure tablets working? 28
Does salt in food affect blood pressure? 28
What about low blood pressure? 28
Taking control of your own blood pressure 28
Key Facts 29

5 ANAEMIA AND ERYTHROPOIETIN

Introduction 30
What is anaemia? 30
Composition of the blood 31
Why do people with kidney failure develop anaemia? 31
Problems with blood transfusions 32
EPO – the 'wonder drug' 32
Who needs EPO? 32
Are there any side effects? 33
Poor response to EPO treatment 33
Anaemia and transplantation 33
Key Facts 34

6 RENAL BONE DISEASE

Introduction 35
Development of renal bone disease 35
What does renal bone disease do? 35
What causes renal bone disease? 35
A combination of causes 36
Parathyroid hormone and kidney failure 36
How is renal bone disease monitored? 37
How is renal bone disease treated? 37
Parathyroidectomy 38
Transplants and renal bone disease 38
Bone pain due to dialysis amyloidosis 38
Key Facts 39

7 BLOOD TESTS AND OTHER TESTS

Introduction 40
The 'figures' 40
Tests for dialysable substances 41
Tests for non-dialysable substances 44
Liver function tests 45
Other blood tests 45
Other tests 46
Finding out about kidney failure 46
Tests for people on dialysis 49
Key Facts 50

8 DIALYSIS – THE BASICS

Introduction 51
What is dialysis? 51
How does dialysis work? 51
The role of the dialysis fluid 51
The dialysis membrane 52
Waste removal by diffusion 52
Fluid removal by ultrafiltration 53
PD or haemodialysis? 54
Key Facts 54

9 PERITONEAL DIALYSIS

Introduction 55
Who can be treated by PD? 55
What does PD do? 55
How does PD work? 55
The peritoneum 56
How is PD done? 56
Operation to insert a PD catheter 57
The training 57
Methods of fluid exchange 58
Fluid exchanges in CAPD 59
Fluid exchanges in APD 59
CAPD or APD? 59
Bigger bags and different types of PD fluid 60
Alternative dialysis fluids 61
Living with PD 61

Delivery and storage of supplies 62
Possible problems with PD 62
Poor drainage 63
Leaks 63
Hernias 63
Peritonitis 64
Exit site infections 64
Key Facts 65

10 HAEMODIALYSIS

Introduction 66
Who can be treated by haemodialysis? 66
What does haemodialysis do? 66
How does haemodialysis work? 66
Different dialysers and machines 67
How is haemodialysis done? 68
'Access' to the bloodstream 68
Fistulas 68
Having 'difficult access' 69
Dialysis catheters 70
Other types of access 70
Single-needle dialysis 71
How much dialysis is needed? 71
Haemodialysis in hospital 72
Satellite haemodialysis 72
Haemodialysis at home 72
Living with haemodialysis 73
Possible problems during haemodialysis 73
Fluid overload and haemodialysis 74
Hyperkalaemia (excess potassium) 74
Problems with access 74
Problems associated with diabetes 75
Bleeding 75
Infections 75
Taking control of your life on haemodialysis 76
Key Facts 76

11 TRANSPLANTATION

Introduction 77
The benefits 77
Who can have a transplant? 77
New kidneys and old diseases 78
Do you have to be on dialysis first? 78
Finding a suitable kidney 79
Matching the blood group 79
Matching the tissue type 79
Testing for viruses 80
Other tests for transplant suitability 80
Cadaveric transplants (and how long they last) 80
Where do cadaveric kidneys come from? 81
Non-heart-beating and living donors 81
Xenotransplantation 81
Stem cell 'kidneys' 82
The transplant waiting list 82
Being ready for a transplant 82
Tests before the operation 83
The transplant operation 83
Key Facts 84

12 LIVING DONOR TRANSPLANTATION

Introduction 85
The benefits (and how long they last) 85
Patient survival after living donor transplants 86
Survival after transplants: comparison to dialysis 87
Cadaveric or living donor transplant – which is best? 87
Who can donate a kidney? 87
Which donor? 88
Who will do the asking? 88
Tests for the recipient 88
Tests for the donor 88
Living unrelated transplants 89
Buying and selling organs 90
Being offered a cadaveric transplant while planning a living donor transplant 90
Preparation for a living donor transplant 90
Removing the kidney from the donor 91

Risks to the donor	91
Risks to the recipient	92
Rejection	92
Conclusion	92
Key Facts	92

13 THE TRANSPLANT OPERATION AND AFTER

Introduction	93
The transplant operation	93
Post-operative tubes	93
After the operation	94
How long will the transplant last?	94
Possible problems after a transplant	96
The rejection process	96
Acute rejection	96
Chronic rejection	97
Immuno-suppressant drugs	98
The 'best' regime of immuno-suppressant drugs	98
Drug side effects	99
Infection	100
Heart disease	100
Cancer	100
Lymphoma	101
Key Facts	101

14 DIET

Introduction	102
Healthy eating guidelines	102
What is 'nutritional status'?	102
Dietary protein and kidney failure	103
Diet before starting dialysis	103
Diet during dialysis	103
Gaining weight (obesity) and kidney failure	103
Losing weight and kidney failure	104
Poor appetite and malnutrition	104
Other causes of weight loss	104
Protein/energy supplements	105
Phosphate and calcium	105
Potassium	105

What about salt and fluid?	106
Vitamin supplements	106
Individual dietary recommendations	106
Diet after a transplant	107
Taking control of what you eat	107
Key Facts	107

15 PSYCHOLOGICAL ASPECTS

Introduction	108
Body and mind	108
Psychological needs	108
Stresses on people with kidney failure	108
The diagnosis	109
Initial reactions	109
Longer-term problems	109
Factors affecting the ability to cope	112
Coping strategies	113
Key Facts	115

16 SEXUAL PROBLEMS

Introduction	116
Investigating sexual problems	116
Erectile dysfunction (impotence)	116
What causes erectile dysfunction?	117
How is erectile dysfunction investigated?	118
How is erectile dysfunction treated?	118
Tablets (Viagra and Cialis)	119
Hormones	119
Vacuum devices	119
Penile injection therapy	120
Penile insertion (transurethral) therapy	120
Penile implants	121
Emotional problems	121
Sexual problems for women	121
Menstrual periods and fertility	122
Pregnancy	123
Key Facts	125

17 DEATH AND DYING

Introduction	126
Death from kidney failure	127
Where should this period be spent?	127
The decision not to start dialysis treatment	127
Trials of dialysis	128
Choosing the lesser of two evils	128
Those who cannot make an informed choice	128
The decision to stop dialysis	129
Withdrawing from treatment after transplant	130
Spiritual concerns	130
Key Facts	131

18 STATISTICS AND OUTCOMES

Introduction	132
Survival with kidney failure	132
Why do people with kidney failure die?	134
Individuals not statistics	135
How good are the services around the world?	136
The 'postcode lottery' in the UK	136
Rate of transplantation	137
Key Facts	138

19 NEW DEVELOPMENTS AND CHOICE

Introduction	139
The number of renal units	139
The number of kidney transplants	139
Choice – real or not?	142
Trying to make it better	143
The Renal National Service Framework	143
Delivering renal services	146
The patients' role in all this	146
Key Facts	147

GLOSSARY	148
FURTHER READING	158
USEFUL ADDRESSES AND WEBSITES	159
INDEX	165
FEEDBACK FORM	175
PRIORITY ORDER FORM	177

FOREWORD

I am delighted to be able to write a Foreword to this 3rd Edition of *Kidney Failure Explained*. The authors, Andy Stein and Janet Wild have improved the book to make it better than ever. Every chapter has been brought right up to date, and they have added a helpful final chapter explaining changes in the NHS which may lead to improving services for kidney patients.

This is quite simply the best book of its kind; the book I recommend to all people I meet who have just found out they have serious kidney disease, and are confronted by so much uncertainty, so much new information, and so many decisions that they do not know where to start. This book packs in a remarkable amount of practical information as well as some complex ideas, and always explains things clearly and simply without ever patronising.

Because it is such a helpful book for people with kidney disease to read, it is of course also very important that all doctors, and other health professionals involved in caring for kidney patients, read it. It will help them with the first and most important art – to communicate with people on their terms, and so help to give them new confidence to keep control of their lives despite all that is happening to them.

John Feehally
Professor of Renal Medicine
Leicester

ACKNOWLEDGEMENTS

Kidney disease is about teamwork. This book could not have been written without the combined efforts of the following people. Professor Gerry Coles (Cardiff) inspired Andy Stein to be a kidney doctor, for which he is thanked. He was subsequently inspired by Dwomoa Adu (QE Birmingham), Tim Mathew (Adelaide, Australia), the late Professor John Walls (Leicester) and Hugh Cairns (King's, London). He has many brilliant current colleagues, especially Rob Higgins and Mair Edmunds, with whom he is honoured to work. John Walls's favourite phrase 'Just Do It' summarises his approach to medicine.

Early in Janet Wild's renal career, she met many enthusiastic people, with most of whom she is still privileged to work. Amongst these are, of course, her co-author and friend Andy Stein whose outlook and attitude to life have made writing so much fun. Donna Lamping, Jean Hooper and Claire Bradley are three psychologists who individually highlighted the importance of good, clear communication and education to Janet. Carina Nilsson, a colleague from Baxter, has continued to coach and inspire her over the years. Ram Gokal, Simon Davies, Edwina Brown and Martin Wilkie are nephrologists who continue to teach, encourage and motivate not only Janet but many other healthcare professionals they meet.

John Walls and Professor Terry Feest (Bristol) were the first doctors to review the first edition of the book, and both devoted much time to improving it. Subsequently the book was also reviewed by Dr Gillian Matthews (Andy's mother), Dr Steve Nelson (St George's, London) and Dr Phin Kon (King's, London). The guest writers, Juliet Auer (Oxford), Gemma Bircher (Leicester), Peter Ellis (King's, London), Jean Hooper (Gloucester), Dr Ian Lawrence (Leicester) and Althea Mahon (Royal London Hospital) all took to their task keenly and with speed. Individual chapters were reviewed by Mr Mark Emberton (UCL), Mr Paul Gibbs (King's, London), Professor John Cunningham (UCL), Professor Mike Nicholson (Leicester), Dr Ian Abbs (Guy's, London), Mr Geoff Koffman (Guy's, London) and Dr Roger Greenwood (Stevenage). For this edition, we are particularly grateful to Professor John Feehally for writing such an encouraging Foreword.

The early force behind the book was Val Said, a kidney patient, who works tirelessly as a volunteer advocate for patients with kidney failure in the UK. Her efforts have been subsequently supported by Austin Donohoe, formerly Chairman of the National Kidney Federation, and by the current chairman Tim Statham OBE.

The publisher, Richard Warner, insisted on literary excellence but never 'pushed' us faster than we could cope with. Darren Bennett is (again) thanked for his clear diagrams and design, and Judith Wise for her tireless work in marketing the book. We also thank Ruth Midgley and Richenda Milton-Thompson, editors of the three editions, for insisting on factual accuracy and clear writing for our readers. They converted this book from something that was 'alright' to something about which we are proud.

This list would not be complete without our thanking our families for supporting us, in particular our partners Emma and Chris.

Andy Stein and Janet Wild

INTRODUCTION

This is a book about kidney failure. It is rare that kidney failure affects only the person who has been given the diagnosis. It affects whole families, friends and work colleagues. The diagnosis can be devastating for those on the sidelines as well as the person in the centre. But, for many people, finding out information and learning to understand their illness can help them get to grips with some of the problems it causes them.

With this in mind we have written a book that we hope will be useful to everyone affected by kidney failure.

I have been involved with the education and training of kidney patients and their families since 1988 and feel strongly that the more you know about your kidney failure, the better you will be able to cope with it. I believe too that no aspect of healthcare is too complicated or difficult to explain. Kidney medicine, along with almost every other medical specialty, is rife with jargon, abbreviations and acronyms. In this book, Andy and I have set out to dispel the myths, unravel the jargon and explain all matters of the kidney as simply and straightforwardly as possible.

The aim therefore is to give you, the reader, the knowledge and confidence to ask questions. This in turn will make it easier for you to get the right information, phrased in the right way. Then you can use this information to make the choices that are best for you, take control of what happens to you and enjoy your life in spite of your kidney failure.

It's often difficult to ask questions in a clinic environment. There isn't always the time and other things often take priority. However, good healthcare is a matter of teamwork. Your healthcare team is not the only team that is important to you. What about your support team at home – your family, friends and colleagues? We have written this book for them as well as for you. The best teams are those in which everyone communicates well with each other, and good communication starts when we all understand what is going on.

As with many other areas of medicine, there are controversies and differences of opinion in the treatment of kidney failure. Andy and I have tried hard to represent the views of the majority and to explain why these disagreements exist. In particular, we discuss a few different ways that are currently used to measure how well your kidneys, dialysis (or a transplant) are working. As this third edition of *Kidney Failure Explained* goes to press, all of the measurements (eg eGFR, creatinine, urea and creatinine clearance) are being used by renal units across the UK. This can be quite confusing, as you may hear one or all of these 'tests' being mentioned by the doctors and nurses at your hospital. We hope that by the time we come to write the next edition of this book, some consensus has been reached and we are able to refer just to one method. We've also included some details of the politics that surround the treatment of kidney failure; the disparities that there are between areas of the UK and the rest of the world. What we hope is that, armed with this information patients can get the best from their own situation and potentially work to improve things for others.

Andy and I remember the dark days before EPO, dialysis being denied to older people, and limited access to APD and living donor transplantation. A lot has changed and improved since then. Even though the disease and its treatment are still tough, there is now hope for you all. This book should maximise that hope, and give you the information you need to get the best healthcare *now* – as well as enabling you to improve care for yourself and others in the future.

Janet Wild

DEDICATION

This book is dedicated to the tens of thousands
of patients with kidney failure in the UK.
Their will to live has inspired us all.

1 WHAT IS KIDNEY FAILURE?

This first chapter begins by explaining how kidneys work. Then it explores what goes wrong when someone has chronic kidney failure, what causes this problem and why it should be treated.

INTRODUCTION

Chronic kidney failure is a serious, long-term medical condition. At the present time, there are approximately 37,400 people in the UK who are either on dialysis or have received a kidney transplant to treat chronic kidney failure. Of these, 40% are on haemodialysis, 14% on peritoneal dialysis (PD) and 46% have a transplant. This is approximately one person in 1,600, making it a rare condition. This means that a typical family doctor will have only one kidney patient 'on their books'.

Chronic kidney failure has many possible causes, but the effects are usually the same. The kidneys become less and less able to do their normal work. After a time, the kidneys stop working almost completely – a condition known as end-stage renal failure (ESRF), end-stage renal disease (ESRD) or end-stage kidney failure. You may hear any one of these titles for kidney failure, but the most widely used term now is established renal failure, or ERF.

There are approximately 6,000 new patients diagnosed with ERF every year.

When the kidneys stop working in this way, trreatment that takes over the work they do becomes essential. The main treatments are dialysis – either peritoneal dialysis (PD) or haemodialysis – and transplantation. These treatments cannot 'cure' kidney failure, but they can improve health and prolong life.

KIDNEYS – WHAT AND WHERE ARE THEY?

Most people have two kidneys. These important body organs are shaped like beans and are about 12 centimetres (5 inches) long, which is about the length of a man's palm. They are approximately 6 centimetres wide and 3 centimetres thick. Each kidney weighs about 150 grams (6 ounces). The kidneys lie under the ribs at the back, just above the waist, one on either side of the body (see *diagram* on next page).

The kidneys lie deep inside the body, so you cannot normally 'feel' them.

THE KIDNEYS' MAIN JOB: MAKING URINE

The main job of the kidneys is to clean up the blood and make urine from the waste products they take out of it. Blood is pumped by the heart to the kidneys. Each kidney has a drainage system that takes urine from that kidney to the bladder. This drainage system is like a funnel with a tube (the ureter) that connects the kidney to the bladder (see *diagram* on next page). Urine passes down the ureters (one for each kidney) into the bladder.

Urine is stored in the bladder before being passed from the body via another tube, called the urethra. The bladder holds about 400 ml (¾ pint) of urine when 'full'.

Location of kidneys and urinary system

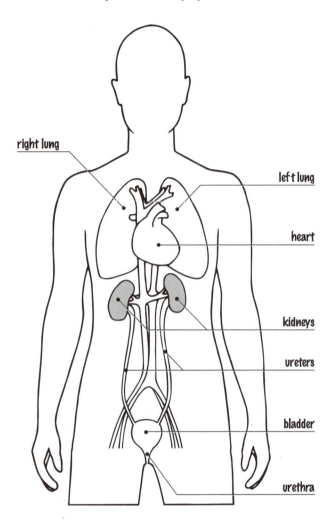

right lung

left lung

heart

kidneys

ureters

bladder

urethra

But when you have just emptied it, by going to the toilet, it will be almost completely empty.

People normally pass around 2 litres (4 pints) of urine per day.

WHY MAKE URINE?

The kidneys make urine in order to perform their two most important functions. These are:

1. Removing toxic wastes from the blood – a process called 'clearance'. (See *below* for a brief description, and *Chapter 2* for more details.)

2. Removing excess salt and water from the body – a process called 'ultrafiltration'. (See *page 3* for a brief description, and *Chapter 3* for more details.)

REMOVING TOXIC WASTES

The kidneys play a very important role in getting rid of waste products. The food we eat is normally digested in the stomach and the bowels. During digestion, the food is broken down into substances that can be carried around the body in the blood. These 'good things' in the bloodstream provide every part of the body with the energy it needs for work, and with the substances necessary for growth and repair.

When the different parts of the body make use of the various 'good things' in the blood, they also produce waste products. These wastes are toxic (poisonous) to the body and make people unwell unless they are removed. Like the 'good things', these 'bad things' also travel around the body in the bloodstream.

When the waste products of food in the blood reach the kidneys, it is the job of the kidneys to get rid of them in the urine. What the kidneys do is to sieve and filter the blood, removing the wastes and putting them in the urine, but leaving the 'good things' in the blood. Healthy kidneys generally have no problems getting rid of all the many toxins normally produced by the body.

In people with kidney failure, however, the levels of toxins build up in the blood. It is this build-up of toxins that makes people with kidney failure feel unwell. When someone is in the early stages of kidney failure, there

A kidney

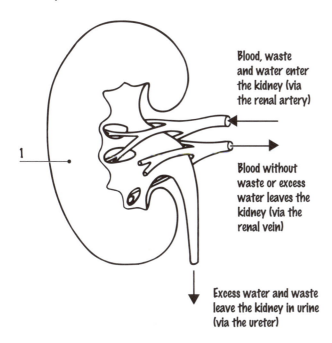

Blood, waste and water enter the kidney (via the renal artery)

Blood without waste or excess water leaves the kidney (via the renal vein)

Excess water and waste leave the kidney in urine (via the ureter)

1 In this part of the kidney there are 1,000,000 filtering units (nephrons)

are usually no symptoms, because the toxin levels are not high enough to cause them. (This can be true even when the kidneys are working at less than 25% of their normal capacity.)

REMOVING EXCESS WATER

The second most important function of the kidneys is to remove excess water from the body. As well as getting rid of the waste products of food, healthy kidneys also remove excess fluids from the body. Like the food that we eat, the water (and tea, coffee, beer and all other liquids) that we drink is digested into the stomach and bowels and absorbed into the blood. When the blood

reaches the kidneys, the normal sieving and filtering process removes any excess water and puts it in the urine. So normal urine contains not only the waste products of food, but also any excess water that has been drunk.

A kidney filtering unit (nephron)

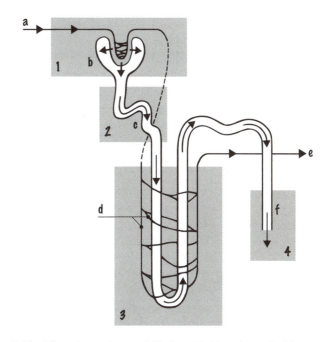

1 Blood from the renal artery (a) is fitered inside a glomerulus (b)

2 Water and waste products filtered from the blood enter a tube system (c)

3 Blood vessels (d) take most of the water back around the body via the renal vein (e)

4 Waste products and excess water (the urine) are removed via a drainage duct (f) that eventually drains into the bladder

In people with kidney failure, water cannot so easily be put into the urine. Excess fluid can therefore build up in the body, causing it to become 'waterlogged' – a condition called fluid overload (see *Chapter 3*). This may lead to swelling of the ankles, and shortness of breath due to excess fluid in the lungs.

OTHER FUNCTIONS OF THE KIDNEYS

As well as water and waste removal, the kidneys have three important 'extra' functions. These are:

1. Helping to control blood pressure. The blood pressure is finely controlled by healthy kidneys. When someone's kidneys fail, their blood pressure usually goes up, although it is not really known why. High blood pressure is unlikely to cause symptoms unless the pressure gets very high, but it increases the risk of a stroke or heart attack, and can cause the kidneys to deteriorate more rapidly (see also *Chapter 4*).

2. Helping to control the manufacture of red blood cells. The kidneys help control the making of red blood cells in the bone marrow (the runny bit in the middle of all bones). The red blood cells float in the liquid part of the blood (called plasma). Their job is to carry oxygen around the body. Every part of the body needs oxygen to function properly.

When someone has kidney failure, they make fewer red blood cells than normal. This causes them to become anaemic (i.e. they are short of red blood cells). This anaemia contributes to the tiredness suffered by most people with kidney failure – it is not only high toxin levels that cause tiredness. (See *Chapter 5* for more about anaemia and how it can be treated.)

3. Helping to keep the bones strong and healthy. Calcium and phosphate are two minerals found in the blood and in the bones. If the bones are to stay strong and healthy, there must be a correct balance between these minerals in the body. The kidneys help to maintain this balance. When someone develops kidney failure, the normal balance between calcium and phosphate in the body is lost. The level of calcium in the blood goes down, while the level of phosphate in the blood goes up. Unless this imbalance is treated, it will result in a condition called renal bone disease. This may cause aches and pains in the bones, and even fractures. (See *Chapter 6* for more information about renal bone disease and its treatment.)

KIDNEY FAILURE – WHAT IS IT?

In short, kidney failure is a condition in which the kidneys are less able than normal to perform their usual functions. These functions are:

- removing toxic waste;
- removing excess water;
- helping to control blood pressure;
- helping to control red blood cell manufacture; and
- helping to keep the bones strong and healthy.

This book is about the long-term condition known as chronic kidney failure or chronic renal failure. There is a separate condition, known as acute kidney failure, in which the kidneys suddenly stop working. Short-term treatment may be needed for acute kidney failure, but the kidneys usually get better on their own. This book does not tell you about acute kidney failure.

When someone's kidneys start to fail, their kidneys become less and less able to do their work. This happens gradually, usually over a period of many years. Eventually, the kidneys stop working almost completely – a condition called established renal failure or ERF. Treatment is then essential to take over the work of the kidneys and so keep the patient alive. The treatments for ERF are dialysis or a kidney transplant (see *page 1*).

WHAT ARE THE SYMPTOMS?

In the early stages of chronic kidney failure, there are often no symptoms. Later, the condition may cause any of the following:

- itching;
- weakness or tiredness;
- loss of appetite;
- poor concentration;
- restless legs;
- leg cramps;
- swollen ankles;
- shortness of breath;
- poor sleeping;
- low sex drive; and
- feeling cold.

HOW IS KIDNEY FAILURE DIAGNOSED?

Kidney failure is diagnosed by measuring kidney function. A reliable way to measure kidney function is to measure the levels of a substance called creatinine in a patient's blood. Creatinine is one of the many waste products that build up in the blood when someone has kidney disease. Many centres then calculate an estimate of kidney function using the serum creatinine and the patient's gender, age and ethnic origin. This is known as an estimated glomerular filtration rate, or eGFR. The eGFR is roughly equivalent to the percentage function the kidney has compared to a healthy kidney.

Creatinine level is measured by a simple blood test. The higher the creatinine level, the worse the kidney function. The normal level of creatinine is between 50 and 120 µmol/l (micromoles per litre of blood), depending on your weight, gender and size.

- **If a person's creatinine is over 120 µmol/l, or their eGFR under 90 mls/min (i.e. 90%), they have kidney failure** (see *Chapter 2*).

As soon as your creatinine level starts to rise, and your eGFR to go below 90, your GP should monitor your health and your kidney function on a regular basis to make sure that serious disease is not beginning to develop.

Creatinine testing is used not only to detect kidney failure, but also used at all stages of kidney disease – before dialysis, during dialysis and after a transplant. The amount of creatinine in the blood is the single most important piece of information that doctors and nurses require when looking after people with kidney failure. (See *Chapter 2* for more information.)

If you have kidney failure, you should know what your blood creatinine level is all the time.

WHAT CAUSES KIDNEYS TO FAIL?

There are hundreds of different diseases that can cause kidneys to start failing, and sometimes to fail completely. Usually, however, ERF (leading to dialysis or a transplant) is likely to be due to one of the following causes:

1. Diabetes mellitus. Diabetes is the most common known cause of kidney failure in the developed world where it may be the cause of ERF in up to 40% of patients in some countries.

Whether diabetes is controlled by insulin, tablets or diet, it can cause kidney failure (known as diabetic nephropathy). This is more likely to happen when someone has had diabetes for more than 10 years. In the UK, an average of 18% of new dialysis patients every year are thought to be suffering from diabetic nephropathy.

The only way of definitely diagnosing this condition is by renal biopsy (see *page 46*). But this procedure carries some risk, so it is not often done.

2. Nephritis. The term 'nephritis' means inflammation of the kidneys ('neph' means 'kidney', and 'it is' means 'inflammation'). The term is usually applied to people with glomerulonephritis or GN. ('Glomerulo' refers to the glomeruli, which are part of the kidneys' filtration unit.)

The causes of most types of nephritis are unknown. Nephritis can only be diagnosed for certain by a kidney biopsy. This involves removing a small piece of kidney to be examined under a microscope (see *page 46*).

3. Polycystic kidney disease (PCKD). This is an inherited disease (a disease that runs in families) in which both kidneys become filled ('poly' means 'many') with cysts (abnormal fluid-filled lumps). If someone has PCKD, they will have a 50% chance of passing the problem on to each of their children.

PCKD is diagnosed by ultrasound (an investigation that uses sound waves to produce a picture of the kidneys). Polycystic kidneys, although abnormally large because of the cysts, do not work well. Many people with PCKD eventually develop ERF.

The cysts in PCKD can remain a problem after treatment for kidney failure has started. A cyst can burst, bleed or get infected – any of which may cause pain. Occasionally, a large cyst that is particularly troublesome will have to be drained through a long, hollow needle inserted into the patient, or removed by an operation. Sometimes, people with polycystic kidneys have to have one of them removed to make room for a transplanted kidney.

4. Pyelonephritis. 'Pyelo' (meaning 'funnel') refers to the drainage system of the kidney and 'nephritis' means 'kidney inflammation', so pyelonephritis means 'inflammation of the kidney drainage system'. Pyelonephritis is diagnosed by ultrasound, or by a special X-ray of the kidneys called an intravenous pyelogram (IVP), in which an opaque dye is injected into the bloodstream. It can also be diagnosed by a special nuclear medicine scan of the kidneys (called a DMSA or MAG-3 scan), in which a small amount of a radioactive substance is injected into the bloodstream.

Pyelonephritis can sometimes be linked to repeated kidney infections. These may have gone undetected for many years, perhaps having occurred in childhood.

Pyelonephritis is sometimes caused by a condition called reflux nephropathy (or 'reflux'). In this condition, a valve where the ureter enters the bladder (see *diagram, page 2*) is faulty. This faulty valve allows urine from the bladder to flow back up the ureter to cause problems in the kidney.

Reflux is a partially inherited condition, particularly in women. So the children of patients with reflux should be tested for it soon after birth. This is true for boys and girls, whichever parent has the condition.

5. Renovascular disease. As people get older, their arteries tend to become 'furred' up with cholesterol and other fats. Smoking makes this process occur at a younger age. This 'furring up' (which is called atheroma or atherosclerosis) gradually narrows the arteries (the blood vessels that take blood from the heart to every part of the body).

Atheroma in the arteries that supply the heart's own muscle leads to angina and heart attacks. If the atheroma affects the arteries that supply blood to the brain, it may cause a stroke. Atheroma can also affect and block the arteries that supply blood to the kidneys, the renal arteries. This is called renovascular disease ('reno' means kidney, and 'vascular' means blood vessel). Renovascular disease is a particularly common cause of kidney failure in older patients. A renal angiogram (see *page 48*) is the only way of definitely diagnosing the condition. But this procedure carries some risk, so it is not often done.

6. Obstructive nephropathy. This is a common cause of ERF in men, especially those over the age of

60 years. It is usually due to enlargement of the prostate gland, which obstructs the urethra (hence the name 'obstructive nephropathy'). The urethra is the tube through which the urine drains from the bladder.

Surgery to the prostate gland (even if it is enlarged due to cancer) can often reverse the kidney failure. But in some cases, especially those cases that were diagnosed late, ERF requiring dialysis will occur even if the patient has had an operation on the prostate to relieve the blockage.

7. Unknown. In about 25% of patients with ERF, the cause of the kidney failure is never discovered. This is because the kidneys often appear small and shrunken when shown by ultrasound. For this reason, a diagnosis of 'two small kidneys' is often made. 'Two small kidneys' really means that the kidneys are small, but doctors don't know why. It is presumed that 'something' happened to the kidneys years ago, and they have slowly shrivelled up since.

THE 'PROGRESSION' OF KIDNEY FAILURE

When chronic kidney failure is still at an early stage, most patients feel quite well. This is because their failing kidneys 'overwork' to keep the level of body waste normal. This hides the fact that the kidneys are failing. In other words, the kidneys have a lot 'in reserve'. The body manages for quite some time to adapt to high levels of toxins and water in the blood. It does this by making the kidneys work harder.

The rate at which kidney failure gets worse varies from patient to patient. Also, the symptoms that patients get when they have similar levels of kidney function can vary considerably. Some patients get symptoms when their kidney function is 70% of normal, whereas others do not get symptoms until their kidney function is down to 5% of normal!

However, for most people with kidney failure, the stages of their kidney failure will be as shown in the table overleaf. Stages 1, 2 and 3 do not necessarily progress to ERF. However, if you are reading this book it is likely that you or someone you care about has Stage 4 kidney failure or worse

If someone has Stage 4 kidney failure – whatever its cause – it is likely that their kidneys will eventually stop working completely. Doctors do not know why failing kidneys usually get worse, or why people with chronic kidney failure usually progress to ERF.

WHAT IS ERF?

This is surprisingly difficult to define. However, most doctors would say that ERF has occurred when treatment by dialysis or a transplant becomes essential for life. When kidney failure is 'established', it very rarely gets better. Once someone develops ERF, they will always have it, even after they have had a transplant (see *Chapter 11*).

If the kidneys start to fail in an older person (say, in someone over 70 years old), that person may live out their natural lifespan without experiencing any problems from their kidneys. This is because the kidneys can take up to 10 years to progress to ERF. So, sometimes, older people never need treatment for their kidney failure. If an older person develops ERF, however, they can still be treated by dialysis or a transplant.

HOW IS ERF TREATED?

ERF can be treated by dialysis or by a kidney transplant. It is usual for a patient to undergo a period of dialysis before transplantation is considered. Dialysis and transplantation provide alternative ways of taking over the work of the patient's failed kidneys.

1. Dialysis. In this treatment, some of the work of the kidneys is performed by artificial means. (See *Chapter 8* for a description of what dialysis is and how it works.) There are two main types of dialysis: PD and haemo-dialysis. (PD is described in detail in *Chapter 9,* and

THE STAGES AND SIGNS OF KIDNEY FAILURE

Stage	Creatinine	eGFR	Dialysis?	Description	Symptoms	Treatment stage	Progression
1	<120	90–99	No	Near-normal kidney function but urine findings or structural abnormalities or genetic traits point to kidney disease	Well	Observation, control of blood pressure and risk factors	May not progress or worsen
2	120–200	60–89	Rarely	Mildly reduced kidney function, and other findings (as for Stage 1) point to kidney disease	Well	No treatment	May not progress
3	200–300	30–59	In 1–5 years, or never	Moderately reduced kidney function	Symptoms variable	Observation, control of blood pressure and risk factors	May progress
4	300–500	15–29	In 3–12 months	Severely reduced kidney function	Unwell	Planning for established renal failure	Usually progresses
5	>500	<15	In less than 3 months	Very severe established or end stage renal failure	Unwell	Treatment choices	Progresses
	>600	<5	Immediate	Life in danger	Severe and unpleasant	Treatment essential	

The Stages 1–5 which form part of this table are based on the KDOQI CKD Guidelines developed in the USA in 2002.

haemodialysis in *Chapter 10*.) Either PD or haemo-dialysis usually provides about 5–10% of the function of two normal kidneys.

2. Transplantation. This treatment involves the removal of a healthy kidney from one person (the donor), and its insertion into a patient with kidney failure (the recipient). Transplantation is done by a surgeon during a transplant operation. A 'good' transplant provides 50–60% of the function of two healthy kidneys. (Transplantation is described in *Chapter 11*.)

WHEN SHOULD DIALYSIS BE STARTED?

Dialysis is usually started either when:

- a patient has symptoms of kidney failure which affect normal daily life; or

- the levels of toxins and/or water in the body are so high that they become life-threatening.

An *eGFR* of 15 mls/minute is generally taken to indicate Stage 5 kidney failure, and the time at which the need for dialysis is becoming imminent. However, the actual level at which dialysis is started varies from patient to patient (*see Chapter 2*). Most doctors now usually try to start patients on dialysis when their eGFR is 5–10 mls/minute, depending on their symptoms. Individual decisions always take into account the patient's condition, and their wishes, not just the eGFR alone.

CAN THE NEED FOR DIALYSIS BE DELAYED?

Once a patient has developed ERF, dialysis should be started very soon. However, if someone with chronic kidney failure has not yet developed ERF, it may sometimes be possible to delay the need for dialysis.

This is particularly true for Stages 1, 2 and 3 of kidney failure, which can often be held 'in check' for years so the patient never progresses to Stage 4 or beyond.

The following treatments may delay the need for dialysis in some patients:

1. Treatments to control blood pressure. High blood pressure is known to speed up kidney failure. Doctors therefore make great efforts to keep the blood pressure of their kidney patients normal. Keeping the blood pressure really low (consistently 130/80 mmHg or less) can delay the need for dialysis by years. This is true for most patients with kidney failure – the cause of the kidney failure makes no difference. (See *Chapter 4* for more about blood pressure and kidney failure.)

2. Treatments to suppress the underlying kidney disease. When kidney failure is due to nephritis (*see page 5*), the need for dialysis can sometimes be delayed by tablets called immuno-suppressants. In some types of nephritis, the body's immune system (the system that normally fights infection or foreign objects in the body) starts to attack the patient's kidneys and stops them working properly. So tablets that make the immune system less effective – such as the steroid tablet called prednisolone – can be used to treat the kidney problem. In some patients, such treatments are very successful, and return the kidney function to normal or near normal. In other patients, these tablets are less successful. Even so, they may delay the need for dialysis by many years. (There is more information on the immune system in *Chapter 14*.)

3. Use of ACE inhibitors/A2-antagonists. This is a more controversial treatment that may delay the need for dialysis in some patients. Some people with kidney failure (especially kidney failure caused by diabetes or nephritis) have a large amount of protein in the urine. Normally, there is next-to-no protein in the urine. If a kidney patient has a raised level of protein in the urine, doctors often attempt to reduce it with a type of blood pressure tablet called an ACE inhibitor or A2-antagonist (also written as AII-antagonist or ARB; or both).

Whether this treatment in fact delays the need to start dialysis is not yet proven.

4. Treating obstructive nephropathy. This is the only cause of ERF that can, in many cases, be wholly or partially reversed. Initially, this is done either by putting a plastic tube (urinary catheter) into the bladder through the urethra; or one or more tubes (nephrostomies) through the skin, into the pelvis (drainage system) of the kidney. Depending on the cause of the obstruction, these procedures in men are usually followed by an operation on the prostate gland, after which the plastic tubes can usually be taken out.

Women do not have a prostate gland, so obstruction in a woman would be caused by something else.

WILL DIALYSIS OR A TRANSPLANT SOLVE THE PROBLEM?

Neither dialysis nor a kidney transplant can 'cure' a patient with ERF. These treatments can control the symptoms of kidney failure, but they cannot get rid of the symptoms completely nor restore the kidneys to health.

1. Dialysis. When someone is treated by dialysis, the symptoms of kidney failure never really go away completely. This is because either type of dialysis – PD (see *Chapter 9*) or haemodialysis (see *Chapter 10*) – can provide only about 5% of the function of two normal kidneys. So when a patient starts dialysis, they will usually have only about 10% of the function of two normal kidneys (5% from dialysis, and 5% from their own kidneys). This is simply not enough to make the person feel completely better. Hence on dialysis the creatinine level usually settles to 500–600 µmol/l before dialysis on haemodialysis, and all the time for patients on PD.

The symptoms of kidney failure will also tend to worsen if the person is not getting enough dialysis. It is important that sufficient dialysis is given to bring the amount of creatinine in a patient's blood down to target level (see *Chapter 2* for more information).

Even though dialysis technology has its limitations, it does do a reasonable job. So it is sensible to start treatment as early as possible – before a patient becomes very unwell. This means that some patients may feel relatively well when they start dialysis. The doctor will be able to tell from a patient's blood creatinine, eGFR and symptoms when is the best time to start dialysis.

2. Transplantation. A kidney transplant is more effective than dialysis at removing the symptoms of kidney failure. This is because a transplanted kidney can provide up to 60% of the function of two normal kidneys. It can be 60% rather than 50% as the new kidney has the potential to grow and overwork. So the patient settles back into Stage 2 kidney failure with a creatinine of 120–200 µmol/l.

However, transplants often have their own problems. They do not last for ever and it may be necessary for a patient to have a second transplant or to resume dialysis if the transplant fails. (See *Chapters 11–13* for more information about transplantation.)

WHY TREAT KIDNEY FAILURE?

If someone with ERF is not treated by dialysis or a transplant, they will develop severe kidney failure symptoms (see *page 5*), and then, after a few weeks, they will die.

Given the terrible result if no treatment is given, it may seem stupid to ask: 'Why treat kidney failure?' The answer seems obvious – 'to keep patients alive'. To a certain extent this is true. When people have ERF, they will die without treatment.

So, certainly, the main purpose of the treatment of ERF is to keep patients alive. However, there is little point in keeping patients alive if their quality of life is so poor that they don't want to be alive.

There are, in fact, several reasons why treatment is given to patients with kidney failure. Firstly, treatment prolongs life in most people. Secondly, it aims to make patients feel better, and to return them to a good quality of life. To achieve this, the two main functions of the kidneys – removing toxins (see *Chapter 2*) and maintaining the body's fluid balance (see *Chapter 3*) – have to be performed for the patient. Dialysis and transplantation can perform both these vital functions.

Doctors are not always sure whether dialysis does actually prolong life for everyone, particularly some people who are both elderly and frail. And if life is prolonged for a short time, there may be costs in terms of the quality of life and the amount of enjoyment the person can get from the extra time. So tablets and injections (e.g. EPO) to control symptoms may be a better option than dialysis for some frail or elderly patients.

5   Many people with chronic (Stage 4) kidney failure will go on to develop ERF, when they will need dialysis or a .

6   For most kidney patients, good control of blood pressure is essential to delay the onset of ERF and the need for dialysis.

7   The treatment of kidney failure (by dialysis or transplantation) is effective, but it is not a 'cure' and may not get rid of all the symptoms.

KEY FACTS

1   The two main functions of your kidneys are:
   - removing toxic wastes;
   - removing excess water and salt.

2   If your kidneys are failing, they will be less able to carry out these functions.

3   Whatever the original cause of your kidney failure, it is likely to get worse over a period of years.

4   A special test (the eGFR) is used to measure the amount of work that the kidneys can still do. This is normally about 100 mls/min, equivalent to 100% of kidney function. If it is less than 90 mls/min (i.e. 90%) you have kidney failure.

2 TOXIN 'CLEARANCE'

This chapter looks at ways of measuring the ability of the kidneys, or dialysis, to remove (or 'clear') waste products or toxins from the blood.

INTRODUCTION

One of the main functions of the kidneys is to remove the toxic waste products of food from the blood. This function is sometimes called 'clearance', because toxins are 'cleared' away. When someone has kidney failure, their kidneys become less efficient at clearing waste products from the blood. This leads to a build-up of toxins in the blood. It is this build-up that makes people with kidney failure feel unwell. Doctors do not know which particular toxin or toxins make people ill.

WHY IS CLEARANCE MEASURED?

Tests that indicate the clearance of toxins from the blood are extremely important when someone has kidney failure.

Clearance measurements are used:

- in the diagnosis of kidney failure;
- to find out how severe the kidney failure is;
- to decide whether it is time for a patient to start treatment by dialysis;
- to monitor treatment by dialysis; and
- to assess how well a transplant is working.

Clearance provides a more reliable guide to a kidney patient's condition than is possible from either a physical examination or an account of the patient's symptoms. Some patients get a lot of symptoms when their kidney function is not too bad. Others get few or no symptoms even when doctors and nurses think that they need dialysis.

HOW IS CLEARANCE MEASURED?

There are tens of thousands of different substances in the blood. Fortunately, there is no need to measure most of them. The overall ability of the kidneys to clear wastes from the blood is assessed by measuring the blood levels of two particular substances. These are called urea and creatinine:

1. Urea is a waste product produced by the liver. When we eat protein (such as in meat and eggs), the body uses this protein (in the form of amino acids) to repair itself and to build muscles. The 'used' proteins are then taken in the blood to the liver, where they are changed into urea. The urea then travels in the blood to the kidneys, where it enters the urine.

2. Creatinine is a substance created by the muscles whenever they are used. The harder our muscles work, the more creatinine they produce. This is a little bit like a car engine producing exhaust fumes. So our muscles are like the engine which drives the car, and creatinine is like the exhaust from the engine. Like urea, creatinine is carried in the blood to the kidneys, where it enters the urine.

Creatinine production

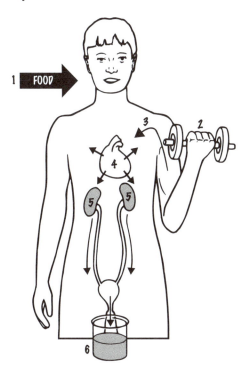

1 Protein is eaten in food
2 Protein is used to make strong muscles
3 Creatinine is produced in the muscles when they are used
4 Creatinine is pumped around the body in the bloodstream by the heart
5 Blood is filtered in the kidneys
6 Creatinine is passed in urine along with other waste products

WHY MEASURE UREA OR CREATININE?

Normal healthy kidneys can remove both urea and creatinine from the body quite well. However, when someone has kidney failure, the blood levels of both these substances rise above normal:

- **The normal blood level of urea** is between 2.6 and 6.6 mmol/l (millimoles of urea per litre of blood).

- **The normal blood level of creatinine** is between 50 and 120 µmol/l (micromoles of creatinine per litre of blood).

Urea and creatinine are not, in themselves, particularly harmful to the body. Creatinine is not even a toxin. However, tests that indicate the clearance of urea and creatinine from the body provide an indication of the clearance of all the thousands of harmful toxins that are produced by the body. In kidney failure, there is a build-up of urea, creatinine and all these toxins.

A substance which is known to indicate the presence of another substance or condition is called a 'marker'. Urea and creatinine do not themselves make people with kidney failure feel ill. However, both urea and creatinine are markers for the many more harmful toxins that do make kidney patients feel ill.

TYPES OF TEST

Different tests show how well or badly the kidneys (or dialysis or a transplanted kidney) are managing to clear the blood of urea or creatinine.

There are basically three types of test:

- **blood tests,** which measure the level of urea or creatinine in the blood (see *page 14*);

- **clearance tests**, which measure the amount of urea or creatinine removed from the blood (see *pages 16–17*);

- **the eGFR,** which measures how many millilitres of blood the kidney is able to filter (and thus 'clean up') in a minute. This gives a good indication of how efficiently the kidneys are working.

BLOOD TESTS FOR UREA OR CREATININE

Blood tests provide a direct measurement of the levels of urea or creatinine present in a patient's blood. These levels can then be compared with normal levels (see *page 13*), or with a range of expected or target levels at different stages of a patient's illness or treatment (see *page 8*).

In simple terms, the higher the levels of urea or creatinine in a patient's blood, the worse the kidney (dialysis or transplant) function. The lower the levels, the better.

In reality, the picture is not quite so simple. Blood urea tests are not always a reliable guide to a patient's kidney function. This is because blood urea levels are affected by things other than the kidneys, such as the amount of protein in the diet. Blood creatinine tests are a generally more reliable guide to kidney function, and have now largely replaced blood urea tests.

It is also the case that blood levels of both urea and creatinine are affected by an individual's overall size and muscle bulk. Larger and more muscular people have higher blood levels of creatinine and urea than smaller and less muscular people. This is true both when someone is healthy and at all stages of kidney failure. Overall size and muscle bulk must therefore be taken into account when looking at an individual's blood urea and blood creatinine test results.

BLOOD CREATININE BEFORE DIALYSIS

Blood tests that measure the level of creatinine in a patient's blood provide doctors with the information they need to decide:

- whether a patient has kidney failure; and

- how bad it is.

The normal level of creatinine in the blood is known to be between 50 and 120 µmol/l. So, if anyone has a creatinine level of over 120 µmol/l, it means that they have kidney failure.

As stated above, the normal level for any particular individual depends on their overall size and muscle bulk. For example, a healthy large man might have a normal blood creatinine of 120 µmol/l (at the top of the normal range). However, the same blood creatinine of 120 µmol/l in a small woman might indicate the start of kidney failure; her normal blood creatinine might be as low as 40 µmol/l (below the bottom level of the normal range).

At the start of kidney failure, the blood creatinine level tends to increase slowly over time. This can take months, or, more often, many years. However, when the kidneys have almost completely failed, the blood creatinine level rises more rapidly. Patients will probably start to feel unwell when their creatinine level gets to more than about 300 µmol/l, equivalent to about 30% of normal kidney function (i.e. chronic kidney failure Stage 4). At a creatinine level of 500 µmol/l (chronic kidney failure Stage 5) almost all patients will feel very unwell.

At all stages of kidney failure, large patients will have a relatively higher blood creatinine than small patients. So, for example, a large man whose kidney function is only 25% of normal could have a creatinine level of 400 µmol/l. A small woman who has 25% of normal kidney function could have a creatinine level of 250 µmol/l.

STARTING DIALYSIS

Dialysis is usually started when a patient's blood creatinine is more than 600 µmol/l. At this stage, the eGFR is likely to be <5 mls/minute (i.e. less than 5% function). Unless someone with kidney failure starts dialysis at this point, they will become very unwell.

The actual creatinine level or eGFR at which any patient starts dialysis will take into account their size and muscle bulk, as well as the degree to which they are troubled by symptoms of kidney failure and feeling generally unwell. Guidelines are based on the needs of an 'average' person, but most people are not average. So the precise levels for starting dialysis are different for different patients.

BLOOD CREATININE DURING DIALYSIS

Measurement of blood creatinine continues to be important after a patient has started dialysis. This applies to patients on either type of dialysis – peritoneal dialysis (PD) (see Chapter 9) or haemodialysis (see Chapter 10).

Blood creatinine level provides vital information about how well dialysis is working. A 'high' level of creatinine could mean that a patient is not getting enough dialysis – i.e. dialysis is not removing enough toxins.

When planning an individual patient's treatment, doctors and nurses aim to keep the patient's blood creatinine at or below recognised 'target' levels. These targets take into account both the size of the patient and the type of dialysis.

The following table summarises the target creatinine levels for different sizes of patient:

Weight	Target creatinine
Less than 60 kg	Less than 500 µmol/l
60–90 kg	Less than 600 µmol/l
More than 90 kg	Less than 800 µmol/l

A blood creatinine of 600 µmol/l is the accepted target level for a person of average size and muscle bulk. As explained below, this target applies all the time for average-sized PD patients, and before dialysis for average-sized haemodialysis patients:

1. PD patients. The blood creatinine of a PD patient remains almost constant. This is because PD patients have dialysis treatment every day. Their treatment therefore aims to keep the creatinine level permanently below 600 µmol/l.

2. Haemodialysis patients. The blood creatinine of a haemodialysis patient does not stay at a constant level. Patients on haemodialysis usually have treatments 2 or 3 times each week. This means that their blood creatinine rises in the days between dialysis sessions, and falls during dialysis. The goal is to keep the creatinine below 600 µmol/l before dialysis, and below 250 µmol/l after dialysis. In other words, a haemodialysis session should cut the creatinine level by at least two thirds.

The fact that the creatinine target levels are the same for PD and haemodialysis (before dialysis) indicates that the two techniques provide roughly the same amount of dialysis. One is not 'better' than the other.

If dialysis does not achieve creatinine target levels over a period of time, the patient will be in danger of, once again, developing the symptoms of kidney failure. This problem is called under-dialysis.

Under-dialysis is corrected by increasing the amount of dialysis. Ways of doing this are described in later chapters (see Chapter 9 for PD, and Chapter 10 for haemodialysis).

BLOOD CREATININE WITH A TRANSPLANT

Ideally, the blood creatinine of an average-sized person with a transplanted kidney should be less than 120 µmol/l (i.e. the upper limit of normal). However, even if a transplant is working well, the blood creatinine may not return to a normal level. This is because the maximum function it can provide is 50–60% of normal.

So the creatinine usually settles settles to around 120–200 µmol/l (i.e. Stage 2 kidney failure). A creatinine level of below 200 µmol/l is generally considered satisfactory for a patient in this situation, so long as it is stable.

If a transplanted kidney starts to fail, the patient's blood creatinine level will rise again. When it exceeds 600 µmol/l, it is probably time to start dialysis again. The creatinine level for restarting dialysis is therefore the same as the level at which a patient who is new to kidney failure would start on dialysis. This is because the period in which a transplant fails is very similar to the period before dialysis is first started.

UREA OR CREATININE CLEARANCE TESTS

Most renal units now use tests called urea or creatinine clearance tests in addition to blood tests for measuring their patients' kidney (dialysis or transplant) function.

Urea or creatinine clearance tests are sometimes preferred to simple blood tests because they link the amount of urea or creatinine in a patient's blood to the size of the patient's muscles. In some situations, this may make these tests a more reliable measure of the severity of a patient's kidney failure.

The test used to measure the clearance of urea is called urea kinetic modelling. The amount of urea clearance is expressed in terms of Kt/V (pronounced 'K...t...over V'). (See *Chapter 10* for more details.)

The clearance of creatinine is measured in millilitres per minute (ml/min) or litres per day (l/d) or week (l/wk).

- **The normal creatinine clearance level** is about 100 ml/min, 150 l/day or 1000 l/wk approx.

A healthy person's blood, therefore, is 'cleaned' about 30 times a day, assuming each person has 5 l of blood.

Blood tests measure the levels of toxins remaining in the blood. So, when blood urea or blood creatinine is measured, the lower the number the better. High numbers reflect poor kidney (dialysis or transplant) function.

The opposite is true for eGFR than for urea and creatinine clearance measurements. Low numbers reflect poor kidney function. This is because clearance (or eGFR) tests measure the amount of toxin *removed* from the blood. So, for clearance test results, the higher the number, the better. A low number indicates poor functioning of the kidneys (or dialysis or transplant).

When the blood creatinine is down to 600 µmol/l (after the onset of ERF), the creatinine clearance is usually down to about 5 ml/min (i.e. about 5% of normal).

Dialysis provides about 5 ml/min of creatinine clearance (i.e. about 5% of normal). So, when a patient starts dialysis, the combined effort of the kidneys and dialysis is only about 10% of what two normal kidneys can do. This is why patients with kidney failure rarely feel perfectly well on dialysis. Neither PD nor haemodialysis is good enough at clearing toxins.

HOW IS CLEARANCE MEASURED?

Different methods for measuring the clearance of urea or creatinine are used for different patients, depending on their type of treatment:

1. Patients not on dialysis. Clearance of urea or creatinine in these patients (either pre-dialysis or with a transplant) is measured by comparing:

- the amount of urea or creatinine passed in the patient's urine over a period of 24 hours; with

- the amount of urea or creatinine in the patient's blood.

To provide accurate results, it is essential that the collection of urine is done very carefully. Every drop of urine collected in the 24-hour period must be collected, otherwise the information will be less reliable than that gained from simple blood urea or blood creatinine tests. Because of this, many doctors now prefer an estimated glomerular filtration rate test or eGFR (see below) that does not need a urine collection.

2. PD patients. The method used for measuring clearance in PD patients is more accurate than that used for patients who are not on dialysis. In PD patients, clearance is measured by comparing:

- the amount of urea or creatinine in 24 hours' worth of the patient's used dialysis fluid, and also in the urine that they might pass; with

- the patient's blood urea or creatinine level (taking into account the patient's size).

3. Haemodialysis patients. For haemodialysis patients, the most accurate method is to compare:

- the patient's blood urea or blood creatinine level before dialysis; with

- the patient's blood urea or blood creatinine level after dialysis.

When measuring clearance in dialysis patients, it is also necessary to take into account patient size, as well as the urea or creatinine passed in any urine after dialysis has been started. Urine production dwindles slowly, making it necessary to increase the amount of dialysis about 1 year after starting dialysis. However, there is some evidence now that the reduction in urine production is slower when patients are having PD than when they are having haemodialysis.

Urea or creatinine clearance during dialysis

When monitoring urea or creatinine clearance in a dialysis patient, doctors and nurses will compare that patient's levels with generally accepted levels for patients on dialysis. The current guidelines state that:

PD patients should have:

- a creatinine clearance of 60 l/wk (litres per week); and

- a urea clearance (Kt/V) of 1.7 l/wk.

Haemodialysis patients should have:

- a creatinine clearance of 100 l/wk; and

- a urea clearance (Kt/V) of 1.2 for each dialysis session.

These goals are the same for all patients as they take into account size and build, as well as the amount of waste that patients can get rid of through their own kidneys.

The eGFR

This test estimates the glomerular filtration rate; the rate at which blood passes through the kidneys in order for the waste products to be extracted. The eGFR is the estimated creatinine clearance of the kidneys.

It is calculated by putting the blood creatinine level into a mathematical equation. This equation makes allowances for the patient's age, sex, weight and race. In this way it 'converts' the blood creatinine level (affected by many other factors) into a percentage of normal kidney function (less affected by those factors).

At present, eGFR is mainly used in the predialysis period.

Different eGFR levels are associated with different stages of kidney failure, as shown in the table on *page 8*.

So, is 'more dialysis' better?

Since the last edition of this book, there has been some important research looking at this question. Studies suggested that, although it was good to give patients the minimum dose (as outlined above), there was no evidence to suggest that 'pushing it' above that minimum dose had any benefits for most patients. Doctors and scientists are still doing research to find out more.

KEY FACTS

1 Creatinine and urea are two waste products that are normally passed in the urine.

2 The levels of urea and creatinine in your blood are an indication of how well the kidneys (or dialysis or a transplant) are working. Blood creatinine level is a more reliable guide than blood urea level.

3 The higher the level of urea or creatinine in your blood, the worse your kidney (dialysis or transplant) function. Generally speaking, the lower the number, the better.

4 The estimated glomerular filtration rate test or eGFR, is now being widely used, either instead of, or in addition to, creatinine clearance tests. Both are used mainly in the predialysis period.

5 This test tells the doctors how well your kidneys are working by measuring the number of millilitres of blood that are cleaned by the filtering system in your kidneys within the space of one minute. It is normally 100 mls/min, which approximates to 100% of kidney function.

6 In contrast to the blood creatinine, the lower the eGFR or creatinine clearance, the worse your kidneys (dialysis or transplant) are working. Generally speaking with these tests, the higher the number, the better.

7 Ideally, dialysis should be started (or a transplant performed) when your creatinine level is 600 μmol/l, or less. At this stage, your eGFR is likely to be less than 5 mls/min (i.e. 5% function).

8 Urea and creatinine clearance tests may be more accurate ways of measuring how well your dialysis is working.

9 Kidney function continues to deteriorate after starting dialysis, making it necessary to increase the dialysis dose, usually after about one year, although this can be sooner for people who have haemodialysis.

10 eGFR, blood creatinine, urea and creatinine clearance are all tests that are used to measure how well your kidneys, dialysis (or a transplant) are working. Different units use different methods. It is not clear yet, which is 'best'.

3 **FLUID BALANCE**

This chapter describes how the amount of water in the body is controlled by the kidneys. It looks at the problem of too much or too little water in the body and gives information on how to deal with it.

INTRODUCTION

One of the two main functions of the kidneys is to remove excess water from the body. Water comes into the body from drinks, and also from food, especially high-liquid food such as soup, jelly and ice-cream. By removing excess water from the body, the kidneys are able to control the body's water content. This is called fluid balance. To understand fluid balance, it helps to know a bit about how the body is made up.

FLESH AND FLUID

The body is made up of two main parts: flesh and fluid. The flesh is all the solid parts of the body, such as bone, muscle and fat. Most of the fluid part is simply water, such as the water in blood, urine and saliva. Men have approximately 60% of fluid to 40% of flesh in their bodies, whereas women, whose bodies contain a higher proportion of fat, have approximately 55% of fluid to 45% of flesh (see *diagram*).

The easiest way to see a change in the amount of fluid in the body is to measure body weight. The known weight of 1 litre of water is 1 kilogram. So, if you weigh yourself, then drink 1 litre of water, then weigh yourself again, your weight will show an increase of 1 kilogram.

Fluid and flesh proportions in the human body

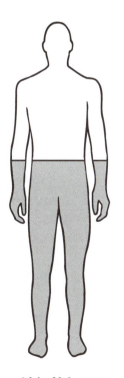

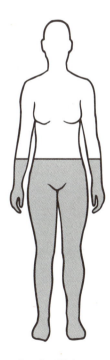

Males 60% water

Females 55% water

WHAT IS THE 'TARGET WEIGHT'?

The term 'target weight' means the weight that the doctor considers to be the 'best' weight for an individual patient. At this weight, there will be neither too much nor too little water in the body. Men will have about 60% fluid to 40% flesh, and women about 55% fluid to 45% flesh. A kidney patient's target weight may have to go up or down as flesh weight is gained or lost. Flesh weight increases if a person eats too much, or may decrease due to dieting or illness.

Weight also changes according to how much fluid is in the body. If a person has too much water in their body (i.e. is fluid overloaded, see below), they will weigh more. The target weight, therefore, is the ideal weight when the person is neither 'wet' (fluid overloaded) nor 'dry' (dehydrated). Sometimes target weight is called 'dry' weight or 'ideal' weight.

Water loss from the human body

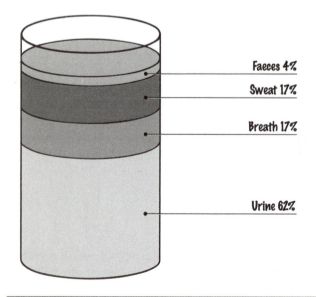

Faeces 4%
Sweat 17%
Breath 17%
Urine 62%

Judging the amount of water in the body is difficult. But with practice, patients can learn to 'feel' when they are at their target weight.

CONTROL OF FLUID BALANCE

Normal healthy kidneys can control the amount of water in the body with ease. If you do not have kidney failure, you do not have to think about your fluid balance because your kidneys control the amount of urine you pass.

If a person drinks 10 pints of water (or beer), they will usually pass about 10 pints of urine. Similarly, if they drink three cups of tea per day, they can expect to pass the equivalent of about three tea cups of urine.

Fluid is also lost from the body in other ways – as you breathe, when you sweat and in your faeces (see *diagram*). If someone becomes very hot, they will sweat more. To control fluid balance, they will then need to compensate for the sweat lost by passing less urine.

In kidney failure, it is different. Many kidney patients do not pass any urine at all. Others pass exactly the same amount of urine every day, no matter how much they drink. This means these patients are unable to control how much water is in the body. If someone with kidney failure drinks too much, they may keep that fluid in their body. This is called fluid overload (see *page 21* for more details). Conversely, if someone with kidney failure drinks too little, or loses too much water from the body (say, through sweating), they will become dehydrated (see *page 21*). Finding the balance is not always easy.

SODIUM (SALT) AND FLUID BALANCE

Sodium is a mineral that plays a part in helping to control the body's fluid balance. Too much of it can contribute to high blood pressure. Table salt contains sodium, so dialysis patients should avoid eating salty foods such as bacon, crisps and many processed foods. They should also avoid adding salt to their food either at table or in cooking. Also, eating salty foods makes people want to drink more fluid. If people with kidney failure drink too much, they may develop fluid overload.

WHAT IS FLUID OVERLOAD?

This is a condition in which there is too much water in the body. It is caused by drinking too much fluid, or not losing enough. Fluid overload often occurs with high blood pressure (see Chapter 4). High blood pressure may not cause any symptoms.

When the water content of the body reaches a very high level, excess water collects in and under the skin. The problem usually first shows as swelling around the ankles. This is called ankle oedema. The reason the ankles are affected first is simple – gravity tends to make fluid fall to the bottom of the body.

If fluid overload is not treated, the swelling due to excess fluid slowly creeps up the body into the thighs, and then into the lower abdomen and lower back. Hopefully, by this stage, the patient will have asked for medical help. If not, fluid will continue to spread up the body, and eventually settle in the lungs. Fluid in the lungs, which causes shortness of breath, is called pulmonary oedema. It is a very serious condition, and can be life-threatening.

Occasionally, people with kidney failure suddenly develop pulmonary oedema, without going through the 'warning stages' of ankle and leg swelling. This can happen if they drink a lot of fluid very quickly. When pulmonary oedema comes on this quickly, it needs urgent treatment. And urgent means exactly that – treatment straight away.

Fluid overload tends to occur mainly in kidney patients on dialysis. However, it can be a problem for pre-dialysis patients too, and also for people who have had a kidney transplant.

HOW IS FLUID OVERLOAD TREATED?

Remember, 'what goes in has to come out'. Therefore the first treatment of fluid overload for all people with kidney failure is simply to drink less. However, this is not usually enough. It is also important that they cut down on salt in their diet, since salt increases thirst. Additional treatments depend on whether or not a patient is on dialysis:

1. In patients not on dialysis. If patients are pre-dialysis, or if they have a failing transplant, they will usually be given tablets called diuretics or 'water tablets' to treat fluid overload. These patients are usually able to pass urine, and the tablets work by increasing the amount of urine that is passed every day. A combination of passing more urine and drinking less usually does the trick. Two commonly used diuretic drugs are furosemide and bumetanide. Stronger diuretics, such as mefruside and metolazone, may be given as well.

If taking diuretics and drinking less does not get rid of all the fluid, it may be necessary to have some dialysis. This may be for just a few days. However, sometimes the difficulty in getting rid of fluid is a sign that kidney failure is well advanced and that dialysis may need to be permanent.

2. In patients on dialysis. Dialysis patients with fluid overload should also drink less. However, because people on dialysis usually pass little urine, diuretics don't normally work for them. A different treatment for fluid overload is needed. These patients need a combination of drinking less (usually a daily limit of 1 litre for haemodialysis patients and 1.5 litres for PD patients), and removing more water by dialysis.

DEHYDRATION

Dehydration is the opposite of fluid overload. It occurs when there is too little water in the body. Dehydration may occur if someone does not drink enough, or if they lose fluid as a result of sweating, diarrhoea or vomiting.

It can be difficult for people to judge when they are dehydrated. However, dehydration is almost always accompanied by low blood pressure. This is easier to identify than high blood pressure. Low blood pressure makes people feel weak and dizzy when they stand up.

HOW IS DEHYDRATION TREATED?

Any patient with kidney failure who is suffering from dehydration needs to drink more.

If a patient (pre-dialysis or with a failing transplant) takes diuretics, these should be reduced or stopped. If the dehydration is severe, admission to hospital for intravenous fluids (via a drip) may be necessary.

For dialysis patients, a reduction in the amount of water removed by dialysis may be needed. If haemodialysis patients are severely dehydrated, they can be given a lot of intravenous fluid during a dialysis session.

TAKING CONTROL OF YOUR OWN FLUID BALANCE

Keeping the right balance of fluid in your body is crucial for long-term health when you are on dialysis. This is particularly important if you have haemodialysis as the dialysis is not done every day and body fluid will build up between treatments.

Keeping the right balance means making sure that the amount you drink is no more than the amount of fluid that is removed by dialysis. You are in control of how much you drink, and can learn to judge how much is safe for you. You can help yourself by not eating salt or salty food, using a small cup to drink out of and spreading your drinks throughout the day. If you get thirsty, sucking an ice cube may help (but don't forget this is water too).

KEY FACTS

1 Fluid balance is the balance between water coming into the body, from drinks and food, and water leaving the body, mainly in the urine or by dialysis.

2 Too much water in the body is called fluid overload. This may cause swelling of the ankles.

3 If you eat salty foods, such as bacon, crisps and many pre-packed foods, you will become very thirsty and will not be able to control your fluid intake. So control of salt intake is vital for control of fluid intake.

4 The treatment of fluid overload is to drink less, and to remove more fluid from the body. This is done by taking diuretics (water tablets), or by increasing the amount of water removed by dialysis.

5 If fluid overload is not treated, shortness of breath due to fluid in the lungs may develop. This condition – known as pulmonary oedema – needs urgent treatment in hospital.

6 Judging the amount of water in the body is difficult. But, with practice, patients can learn to 'feel' when they are on their target weight – i.e. when they are neither 'wet' (fluid overloaded) nor 'dry' (dehydrated).

7 When there is too little water in the body (dehydration), dizziness may occur.

8 The treatment of dehydration is to drink more, and to remove less water from the body. This is done either by stopping diuretics, or by reducing the amount of water removed by dialysis.

9 Fluid balance is one area where you can really take control and do a lot to help yourself. Make sure that the amount you drink is no more than the amount of fluid that can be removed by dialysis, and learn to judge how much is safe for you. Help yourself by avoiding salty food (that makes you thirsty), using a small cup to drink out of and spreading your drinks throughout the day.

4 BLOOD PRESSURE

This chapter looks at the link between blood pressure and kidney failure. It also explains the importance of blood pressure control and how this is achieved.

INTRODUCTION

The control of blood pressure is one of the important 'extra' functions performed by the kidneys. The term 'blood pressure' means the pressure of the blood on the artery walls. This pressure goes up and down as the heart continuously squeezes and relaxes to pump blood around the body. Although the kidneys are known to help control the blood pressure, exactly how they do this is not clearly understood.

HIGH BLOOD PRESSURE AND KIDNEY FAILURE

High blood pressure is very common in people with kidney failure. The connection between these two conditions is two-way. High blood pressure can cause kidney failure, and kidney failure causes high blood pressure. It is often difficult to know for certain whether a patient's high blood pressure has caused their kidney failure, or whether kidney failure has caused their high blood pressure.

High blood pressure can occur in kidney patients who are pre-dialysis, who are on dialysis, or who have had a transplant. Many patients with kidney failure are taking one, two or even three types of blood pressure tablet.

Many patients with kidney failure have to take an injection treatment called erythropoietin (EPO) for anaemia. If you have high blood pressure, this treatment

can make it worse. It is better, however, to stay on the drug if you need it, and to take more blood pressure tablets, than to stop EPO.

LOW BLOOD PRESSURE AND KIDNEY FAILURE

Some people with kidney failure have a different blood pressure problem. Their blood pressure is lower than it should be. Low blood pressure is usually less serious than high blood pressure, but it also needs to be treated.

Very low blood pressure can be serious though. It can be a sign that the heart is not pumping well (heart failure).

CIRCULATION OF THE BLOOD

The main function of the blood (and the blood vessels through which it flows) is to carry things around the body. Blood carries 'good things' to parts of the body where they are needed, and also removes 'bad things' so they can be got rid of, mainly by the kidneys via the urine.

Adults have about 5 litres (10 pints) of blood travelling around their body all the time. The heart acts as a pump to drive the blood through the blood vessels. There are two main types of blood vessel: arteries and veins. The arteries take blood that is rich in oxygen from the heart to all parts of the body. This oxygen, combined with the

Circulation of blood in the human body

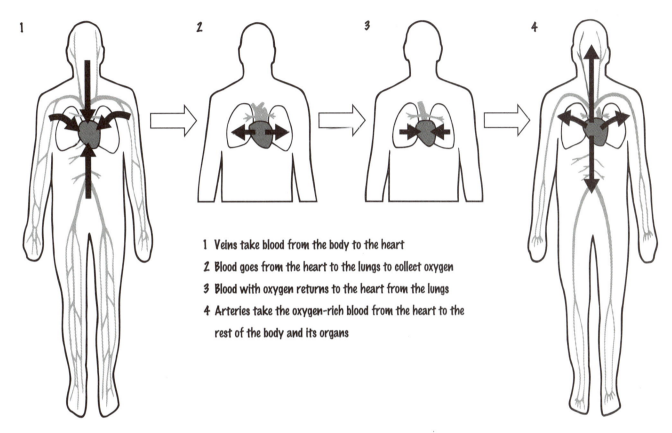

1 Veins take blood from the body to the heart

2 Blood goes from the heart to the lungs to collect oxygen

3 Blood with oxygen returns to the heart from the lungs

4 Arteries take the oxygen-rich blood from the heart to the rest of the body and its organs

food that is eaten, provides the different parts of the body with the energy they need to do their work. The veins then take the blood (now with most of its oxygen used up) back to the heart. From there, the blood goes to the lungs to get more oxygen. It then goes back to the heart, and so the process goes on (see *diagram* above).

MEASURING BLOOD PRESSURE

The blood pressure is measured using a piece of equipment known as a sphygmomanometer (or sphyg, pronounced 'sfig'). There are various different types of sphygmomanometer, but all of them measure blood pressure in units of millimetres of mercury (mmHg).

Two readings are taken. The first reading shows the pressure of the blood when the heart squeezes, and is called the systolic blood pressure. The second reading is the pressure of the blood when the heart is relaxed between squeezes. This is called the diastolic blood pressure.

The systolic pressure is always higher than the diastolic pressure, and is always recorded first. So, for example, a blood pressure of 140/80 mmHg (known

Blood pressure

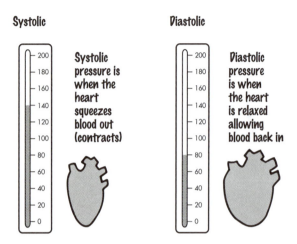

Systolic

Systolic pressure is when the heart squeezes blood out (contracts)

Diastolic

Diastolic pressure is when the heart is relaxed allowing blood back in

as '140 over 80') means that the systolic pressure is 140 and the diastolic pressure is 80.

A reading of 140 mmHg means that the blood pressure has raised the top of the mercury (Hg) column inside the sphygmomanometer to a height of 140 millimetres.

WHAT IS 'NORMAL' BLOOD PRESSURE?

There is no such thing as normal blood pressure. Both the systolic and the diastolic blood pressure go up naturally as people get older. So there is only a normal *range* of blood pressure for your age. Most doctors accept the following values as the normal range for different age groups:

Age Group	Blood Pressure (in mmHg)	
	Systolic	**Diastolic**
Under 30 years	100–120	60–70
30–60 years	110–130	70–80
Over 60 years	120–140	80–90

For most people with kidney failure, however, doctors accept a level of 130/80 or below as satisfactory. This is for patients who are not yet on dialysis, those on PD or with a transplant, or before a haemodialysis session.

The blood pressure varies continuously throughout the heart's pumping cycle. This means that during each cycle, the systolic blood pressure is, say, 140 or 180 for only a fraction of a second.

Blood pressure also varies according to the time of day – tending to be higher in the morning and again in the early evening. And there is a difference between one arm and the other. Slight variations may also result from using different sphygmomanometers, or from how different people use the same piece of equipment.

If there is doubt about whether or not a patient has high blood pressure, a 24-hour blood pressure test can be organised. This involves a patient carrying a cuff on their arm for 24 hours. Every hour, the cuff automatically inflates and deflates, giving the doctor a better idea of the average blood pressure over the 24-hour period.

DOES ANXIETY AFFECT BLOOD PRESSURE?

Anxiety is definitely not a major factor in high blood pressure. Although anxiety can put the blood pressure up a little, it is a mistake to blame repeated high blood pressure readings on, for example, 'the stress of the journey' or a 'fear of seeing the doctor', or even 'difficulty parking'.

HOW DO YOU KNOW THAT YOUR BLOOD PRESSURE IS HIGH OR LOW?

You don't. Some people with very high blood pressure suffer from headaches. But the fact that you do not have headaches does not mean that you do not have high blood pressure. The only reliable way of finding out what your blood pressure is, is to have it measured.

If your blood pressure is very low, you may feel weak or dizzy, especially when you stand up. But there are many other causes of weakness and dizziness. So, as with high blood pressure, you cannot rely on your body to tell you that your blood pressure is low. You have to have your blood pressure checked.

WHY TREAT HIGH BLOOD PRESSURE?

There are several important reasons to treat high blood pressure (see *overleaf*). However, there is little point in treating someone for high blood pressure unless the related problems of high cholesterol levels in the blood, being overweight and smoking are also addressed. All these factors worsen the effects of high blood pressure.

High blood pressure increases the likelihood of a stroke or a heart attack by damaging the blood vessels. There are also 'kidney reasons' to treat high blood pressure. If blood pressure is high for a period of time, a patient with kidney failure may have to start dialysis sooner than would otherwise be necessary. This is because uncontrolled high blood pressure can accelerate kidney failure.

In fact, controlling blood pressure is the only thing proven to delay the need for dialysis in all kidney patients, whatever the cause of their kidney failure. Good blood pressure control does not mean they will never need dialysis, but it may mean that dialysis does not need to be started so soon. It may also prolong the life of a transplant.

WHAT DETERMINES BLOOD PRESSURE LEVELS?

A person's blood pressure is affected by the following important factors:

1. The amount of water in the body. If there is too much water in the body (fluid overload), the blood pressure will go up. If there is too little water in the body (dehydration), the blood pressure will go down. (Both fluid overload and dehydration, and their treatments, are described in *Chapter 3*.)

2. The width of the arteries. The arteries are constantly changing in width as blood flows through them. The narrower the arteries, the higher the blood pressure.

3. The heart (the pump). The strength of contraction of the heart, and the rate it beats, also affect blood pressure. Generally speaking, the harder or faster the heart beats, the higher the blood pressure will be.

HOW IS HIGH BLOOD PRESSURE TREATED?

Because there are 3 main factors contributing to high blood pressure, there are also 3 different ways of treating it:

1. By reducing the amount of water in the body. If someone has fluid overload, their blood pressure will increase. This is because their blood contains more water than normal, which increases the pressure on the blood vessels. Correcting fluid overload (see *Chapter 3*) with diuretics (water tablets) or dialysis will reduce the blood pressure. Eating a lot of salty foods and adding extra salt to meals makes people thirsty and leads to them drinking more (see *page 21*). So people with kidney failure should cut down on salt as well as fluid.

2. By increasing the width of the arteries (with vasodilator drugs). Blood pressure tablets called vasodilators lower the blood pressure by causing the arteries to widen. There are several different types of vasodilator drug:

- ACE inhibitors (e.g. captopril, enalapril, lisinopril, perindopril and ramipril);

- alphablockers (e.g. doxazosin, prazosin and terazosin);

- calcium antagonists (e.g. amlodipine, diltiazem, felodipine and nifedipine);

- angiotensin II antagonists (e.g. candesartan, irbesartan, losartan, telmisartan); and

- other tablets (e.g. hydralazine, methyldopa, minoxidil and moxonidine). Minoxidil is probably the strongest drug available, and can be extremely useful for kidney patients with very high blood pressure.

3. By decreasing the strength of contraction of the heart, and the rate at which it beats (using beta-blocker drugs). These tablets reduce the force of contraction and the heart rate (the number of heart beats per minute). They also lower the blood pressure, although how they do this is not clear. Commonly used examples of beta-blockers are atenolol, bisoprolol, carvedilol, labetalol, metoprolol and propranolol.

ARE THE BLOOD PRESSURE TABLETS WORKING?

As blood pressure has to be very high before it causes symptoms (such as headaches), most people cannot 'feel' that their blood pressure is raised. Not surprisingly, therefore, they also cannot tell whether or not their blood pressure tablets are working. The only reliable way of knowing a person's blood pressure, and discovering whether it is responding to tablets, is for the blood pressure to be measured.

DOES SALT IN FOOD AFFECT BLOOD PRESSURE?

Too much sodium (salt) in the body can increase the blood pressure. This is because a salty diet makes people thirsty and encourages them to drink more. However, salt is not the only thing that causes high blood pressure (see page 27). People who have high blood pressure will be asked to eat less salt and take tablets to help keep it under control.

WHAT ABOUT LOW BLOOD PRESSURE?

Low blood pressure is not as common as high blood pressure. It is normally less serious and easier to treat. This is partly because people can often feel that their blood pressure is low. So they can also feel when it is back to normal.

Low blood pressure in people with kidney failure is usually due either to dehydration, or to taking too many blood pressure tablets. Therefore, the treatment is either to drink more to correct the dehydration, or to alter the dose of blood pressure tablets or stop the tablets.

TAKING CONTROL OF YOUR OWN BLOOD PRESSURE

High blood pressure is not something you just need to 'suffer' with. The three golden rules for keeping your blood pressure down are:

- take your blood pressure tablets;

- don't get fluid-overloaded;

- don't eat too much salt.

KEY FACTS

1 High blood pressure is very common in people with kidney failure.

2 An acceptable blood pressure will be 130/80 or below, for most people.

3 Kidney failure causes high blood pressure, and high blood pressure causes kidney failure.

4 The injection treatment for anaemia, called erythropoietin (or EPO), can increase your blood pressure.

5 High blood pressure also increases the likelihood of a stroke or heart attack.

6 You cannot reliably 'feel' your own blood pressure, especially when it is high. You have to have it checked.

7 High blood pressure can be controlled by removing fluid from your body and by taking blood pressure tablets.

8 Too much salt in the diet may make the blood pressure higher.

9 You have the opportunity to take a large part of responsibility for controlling your own blood pressure. Have it checked regularly, don't drink too much fluid, avoid salt wherever possible, and make sure you take the tablets your doctor prescribes for you.

5 ANAEMIA AND ERYTHROPOIETIN

This chapter explains what anaemia is, and how the drug erythropoietin (EPO) has revolutionised its treatment. EPO is probably the most important drug taken by patients who need it.

INTRODUCTION

Many patients with kidney failure have a condition called anaemia. This means that they have a lack of red blood cells in their body. Blood cells are produced in the bone marrow, the 'runny' bit in the middle of the bones. An important 'extra' function of the kidneys is to help control the manufacture of red blood cells in the bone marrow.

WHAT IS ANAEMIA?

Anaemia is the term for a lack of red blood cells in the body. The main symptoms are tiredness, shortness of breath, pale skin, poor appetite, irritability and low sex drive. Anaemia is probably the most important complication of kidney failure. It is the main reason why dialysis patients feel weak and tired. In fact, many of the symptoms of kidney failure are not caused by kidney failure itself, but are actually due to anaemia.

Red blood cells are needed to carry oxygen around the body. Oxygen enters the lungs when we breathe in. From the lungs, oxygen is taken around the body in the blood. Each red blood cell contains a substance called haemoglobin. It is the haemoglobin that carries oxygen around the body. Oxygen combines with the nutrients taken in from food to provide energy.

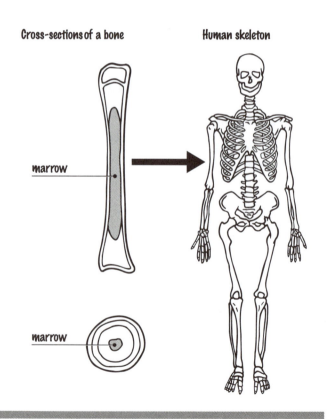

Location of bone marrow

Cross-sections of a bone

Human skeleton

marrow

marrow

Measuring the level of haemoglobin (or 'Hb') in the blood provides a guide to the number of red cells present. The higher the Hb, the more red blood cells there are in the body. As it is red blood cells that are able to carry oxygen round the body, in general the higher the Hb the better (but see *page 32*).

Normal Hb levels are 12–17 g/dl (grams of haemoglobin per decilitre of blood).

- **If your Hb is below 11 g/dl, you have anaemia.**

COMPOSITION OF THE BLOOD

Blood is made up of two parts: a liquid part and a more solid part. The liquid part is called plasma. It accounts for about 60% of the blood's volume, and is mainly water. The amount of water in the plasma is increased in fluid overload and decreased in dehydration. (Both these conditions were described in *Chapter 3*.)

The other 40% of the blood is made up of blood cells, which are so tiny that they can only be seen through a microscope. There are various different types of cells: red cells (which carry oxygen around the body), white cells (which fight infection) and platelets (involved in blood clotting). Most of the blood cells are red cells. It is these cells that give the blood its red colour. Each one looks rather like a tiny doughnut. Red cells are smaller than white cells, and larger than platelets. You have about 5 billion red cells in one drop of blood.

WHY DO PEOPLE WITH KIDNEY FAILURE DEVELOP ANAEMIA?

The main reason that kidney patients develop anaemia is this. One of the jobs the kidneys do, in addition to their main job of making urine, is to manage the production of red blood cells in the bone marrow. To do this, the kidneys make a substance called erythropoietin (EPO).

EPO travels in the blood from the kidneys to the bone

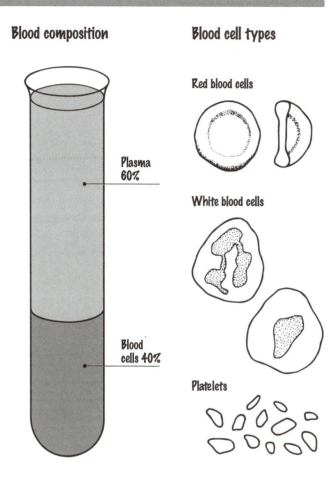

Blood composition

Plasma 60%

Blood cells 40%

Blood cell types

Red blood cells

White blood cells

Platelets

marrow, where it constantly reminds the bone marrow to keep producing red cells. When someone has kidney failure, the kidneys usually make less EPO than normal. So the bone marrow 'goes to sleep' and makes fewer red cells. As a result, anaemia develops, and the patient becomes weak and tired.

Some patients with kidney failure develop anaemia even though their EPO level is normal (or even high). This probably means that their bone marrow has a problem reacting to EPO, rather than that the kidneys are not making enough EPO. Although a lack of EPO is the main cause of anaemia in people with kidney failure, other things may contribute. For example, red blood cells do not live as long as normal (120 days) in people with kidney failure, and so must be replaced more rapidly. Also, blood may be lost during haemodialysis, or through frequent blood tests.

PROBLEMS WITH BLOOD TRANSFUSIONS

In the past – before the introduction of EPO injections (see *below*) – blood transfusions were the only treatment for anaemia in kidney patients. Many patients had to have transfusions every couple of months, since each transfusion could improve anaemia for a few weeks only.

Blood transfusions can cause serious problems for patients on dialysis. These include fluid overload (see *Chapter 3*), and the storage of surplus iron in the liver (which can lead to liver failure). Another problem is that whenever a transfusion of blood is received, the body produces substances called antibodies. These antibodies stay in the blood for years and can cause problems if the patient is then given a transplant. The antibodies can attack (and cause the body to reject) the new kidney.

The risk of contracting hepatitis B, hepatitis C or HIV (the virus that causes AIDS) from a blood transfusion is small in the UK. Even so, if someone does not need a blood transfusion, it is better not to have one.

Blood transfusions are still sometimes needed by kidney patients – for example, after severe bleeding. In general, however, treatment with EPO has turned regular blood transfusions into a thing of the past for kidney patients.

EPO – THE 'WONDER DRUG'

Synthetically produced EPO became available as an injection in the late 1980s – probably the most important advance in the treatment of patients with kidney failure. In 2004, 91% of haemodialysis patients and 77% of PD patients were on EPO. This is because patients on PD tend to have less of a problem with anaemia. If they are prescribed EPO, they usually need a lower dose.

EPO works well in most patients, and usually gets rid of the tiredness and other symptoms caused by anaemia.

EPO is generally given in the form of an injection under the skin (called a subcutaneous injection). This is needed one to three times a week, though there is a newer form of EPO called darbepoetin alfa (Aranesp) which can be given less frequently than traditional EPO (sometimes every 2 weeks). Some patients may be asked to give their own injections. The aim of the treatment is to raise the Hb level in the blood to between 11 and 12 g/dl. Without this treatment, most patients with kidney failure will have an Hb between 6 and 8 g/dl.

A patient's response to EPO depends on how much they are given. The higher or more frequent the dose, the higher the patient's blood Hb level will go. However, there is no point in making the Hb go above 12 g/dl – the patient will feel no better. In fact, problems may occur if the Hb goes over 14 g/dl. So, the target Hb is 11–12 g/dl in most patients, and they should take EPO only as prescribed.

WHO NEEDS EPO?

Patients who are on dialysis – either PD (see *Chapter 9*) or haemodialysis (see *Chapter 10*) – often need EPO. But, for most patients, anaemia actually begins long before they need to start dialysis. Therefore many doctors now give EPO before the start of dialysis, in the predialysis period. Transplant patients should also be considered for EPO if their Hb falls below 11 g/dl, especially if the transplant is failing, as anaemia often returns at this time. However, there are some doctors who prefer to delay starting treatment with EPO until 3 months after the start of dialysis. This is because the start of dialysis will sometimes 'cure' a patient's anaemia – perhaps because dialysis removes toxins that may interfere with the way the bone marrow works.

Treatment with EPO has been found to be very useful even in those kidney failure patients who have anaemia without having a reduced EPO level. It is not known why giving very high doses of EPO to these patients should make such a difference to their anaemia, but it does.

Some patients with kidney failure – especially those with polycystic kidney disease (see *page 5*) – do not become anaemic, as their kidneys continue to produce EPO, even when on dialysis. They therefore do not usually need EPO treatment.

ARE THERE ANY SIDE EFFECTS?

The only common side effect of EPO is worsening of high blood pressure. This is most likely in patients who have had severe high blood pressure in the past, or in patients who are on more than one type of blood pressure tablet. If the blood pressure does increase, more blood pressure tablets may need to be taken. A combination of EPO and high blood pressure can sometimes cause epileptic fits, but this problem can usually be prevented by treating the high blood pressure.

POOR RESPONSE TO EPO TREATMENT

Most, but not all, patients respond to regular treatment with EPO. However, EPO may not work if other conditions are present. These include infections – especially repeated peritonitis in PD patients, and dialysis catheter site infections in haemodialysis patients. It also may not work if there is under-dialysis (failure of dialysis to achieve target creatinine and urea levels), renal bone disease (see *Chapter 6*) or iron deficiency.

Iron deficiency is the most common reason for EPO not to work. EPO causes the body's iron stores to be used up more quickly than usual. In an attempt to spot the onset of iron deficiency, patients are given regular blood tests to measure a substance called ferritin (see *page 46*). Blood ferritin levels provide a guide to the amount of iron stored in the body and low levels of ferritin indicate iron deficiency.

If iron deficiency is discovered, the doctors should investigate *why* the patient lacks iron. One important cause could be bleeding (that may not have been noticed by the patient) from somewhere in the bowel.

If such causes of iron deficiency can be ruled out, it can sometimes be treated with iron tablets (usually a type called ferrous sulphate). Other patients need regular iron injections. These days, iron injections rather than tablets are usually given.

If EPO stops working – for whatever reason – the Hb will return to the 'normal' low level in people with kidney failure (usually 6–8 g/dl). The symptoms of anaemia will then return.

ANAEMIA AND TRANSPLANTATION

After a kidney transplant, the new kidney will start making EPO for the patient and the problem of anaemia usually goes away. Injections of EPO will then no longer be needed. However, if the transplanted kidney ever fails, anaemia will usually return, and EPO injections may be needed again.

KEY FACTS

1 Many patients who have kidney failure (predialysis, on dialysis or with a transplant) have a condition called anaemia. This means you have a lack of red blood cells.

2 Anaemia is the main reason why dialysis patients are weak and tired.

3 The severity of anaemia is measured by a blood test called a haemoglobin (or 'Hb') test.

4 If your Hb is below 11 g/dl, you have anaemia.

5 The lower your Hb level, the more anaemic and tired you will be.

6 Anaemia is easy to treat with injections of substances called erythropoietin (EPO; called Neorecormon or Eprex) or darbepoetin alfa (Aranesp).

7 All patients (predialysis, on dialysis or with a transplant) with an Hb below 11 g/dl should be considered for EPO. The target Hb is 11–12 g/dl in most patients.

8 Patients on EPO treatment may need additional iron in the form of either tablets or injections.

9 EPO is very good at controlling symptoms and giving you more energy. You should only stop taking it or miss a dose if your kidney doctor tells you to.

10 If you have a transplant that is working well, you can usually stop taking EPO.

6 RENAL BONE DISEASE

This chapter provides information on the causes, prevention and treatment of renal bone disease (also known as renal osteo-dystrophy), which is a common complication of kidney failure.

INTRODUCTION

Most people with kidney failure have some degree of renal bone disease. This is because one of the 'extra' functions of the kidneys is to help make the bones strong and healthy. For the bones to be strong, the kidneys must be able to maintain a healthy balance of various substances – including calcium, phosphate and vitamin D – in the body. Kidney failure results in abnormal levels of these substances, and so leads to renal bone disease.

DEVELOPMENT OF RENAL BONE DISEASE

Blood tests will reveal abnormal levels of calcium, phosphate and vitamin D in a patient's blood very early in kidney failure, long before dialysis is required. The calcium and vitamin D levels will be lower than they should be, while the phosphate level will be too high. These changes can be seen in Stage 2 of chronic kidney failure (i.e. 60–90% kidney function).

Abnormalities in calcium, phosphate and vitamin D levels do not usually lead to problems that a patient is likely to notice until after the start of dialysis. However, treatment should be started at an early stage to prevent weakening of the bones. This may also help prevent problems with the heart.

WHAT DOES RENAL BONE DISEASE DO?

Without treatment, renal bone disease can lead to pain in the bones, especially in the back, hips, legs and knees. The weakened bones also become increasingly prone to fracture. The heart can also be affected. However, early recognition and treatment of renal bone disease means that bone pain and fractures are now uncommon in kidney patients.

WHAT CAUSES RENAL BONE DISEASE?

There are three main causes of renal bone disease:

1. Low calcium levels in the blood. Calcium is a mineral that strengthens the bones. It is obtained from some foods, especially dairy products, eggs and green vegetables. In our bodies, calcium is stored in the bones. There is also some calcium in the blood. The kidneys normally help to keep calcium in the bones. In people with kidney failure, calcium drains out of the bones and is lost from the body. This leads to a fall in the level of calcium in the blood.

The normal blood calcium level is between 2.1 and 2.6 mmol/l (millimoles per litre of blood). In kidney patients, the level of calcium in the blood may fall below 2.0 mmol/l. Treatment can keep the calcium level up quite easily.

2. High phosphate levels in the blood. Phosphate is another mineral that strengthens the bones. Foods that contain phosphate include dairy products, nuts and meat. Like calcium, phosphate is stored in the body in the bones and is also present in the blood. The kidneys normally help to keep the right amount in the blood – not too much, not too little. In people with kidney failure, phosphate builds up in the blood.

The normal level of phosphate in the blood is 0.75–1.4 mmol/l. In kidney patients, it is common for the blood phosphate level to be high, rising to more than 2.0 mmol/l. Unfortunately, it is quite difficult to keep phosphate levels normal. High phosphate levels are thought to cause itching.

3. Low vitamin D levels in the blood. Vitamin D is needed in the body so that calcium from the diet can be absorbed into the body and used to strengthen the bones. Vitamin D is found in some foods, especially margarine and butter. However, most of our vitamin D is made by the skin (a process that only occurs if the skin is stimulated by sunlight). Unfortunately, vitamin D from food and from the skin are in a form which the body cannot use directly. The kidneys are responsible for transforming vitamin D into a usable substance.

Blood levels of the usable form of vitamin D are not usually measured, as the blood test is expensive and difficult to do. If they were measured, they would be low. It is quite easy to provide additional vitamin D as tablets or injections, although not all kidney patients need it. Often, it will be enough just to control the levels of calcium and phosphate.

A COMBINATION OF CAUSES

Doctors do not know which of the three main causes of renal bone disease comes first. Nor do they know what leads to what. They do know, however, that although any one of these causes can lead to problems, a combination of the three is usually present in people with kidney failure. More importantly, each of the causes tends to have a 'knock-on' effect, worsening the other two abnormalities. For example, a high phosphate level tends to lower the calcium level, and vice versa. It is important, therefore, to treat all three causes (see *page 37*).

PARATHYROID HORMONE AND KIDNEY FAILURE

Parathyroid hormone (PTH) is a substance produced by four tiny glands called the parathyroid glands. These glands are situated in the front of the neck (see *diagram*). Normally the parathyroid glands (and the kidney) keep calcium, phosphate and vitamin D levels in balance. When someone has kidney failure, however, the parathyroid glands become overactive and produce too much PTH, and renal bone disease starts.

Location of the parathyroid glands

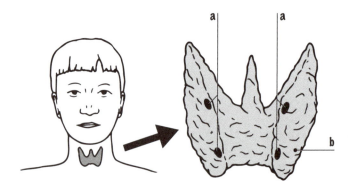

The parathyroid glands (a) are four tiny glands located at the back of the thyroid gland (b), in the neck

HOW IS RENAL BONE DISEASE MONITORED?

The levels of calcium and phosphate in a kidney patient's blood can tell us what is happening in the bones at the time of the test. However, these levels provide little information about the future.

The best guide to the progress and severity of renal bone disease is the amount of PTH in the blood. PTH tells us much more about the long-term health of the bones. Changes in blood PTH can tell us about what will happen to the bones in the future – the lower the PTH, the better.

Renal bone disease begins very early in kidney failure. It is therefore a good idea for doctors to measure a patient's blood PTH even before dialysis is necessary. Once dialysis has started, most doctors should measure the blood PTH at least every 3 months. A high level (i.e. greater than 20 picomoles per litre of fluid) indicates a problem with the bones. Doctors will then start a range of treatments to help prevent any worsening of the problem. Even very high PTH levels can usually be lowered with the right tablets.

The target PTH level is less than twice the upper limit of normal (normal is 1.1–4.2 pmol/l). So a PTH level of less than 10 pmol/l is considered satisfactory.

HOW IS RENAL BONE DISEASE TREATED?

Treatment may be needed for each of the three main causes of renal bone disease. All patients with kidney failure, whether they are predialysis, on dialysis or with a transplant, have some degree of renal bone disease. Most will require treatment.

1. Raising low calcium levels. Patients on dialysis can obtain some extra calcium from the dialysis fluid. This happens because there is more calcium in some dialysis fluids than there is in the blood. Calcium passes from the stronger solution (the dialysis fluid) into the patient's blood (the weaker solution) by a process called diffusion. (See *Chapter 8* for more information on diffusion.)

For many kidney patients, extra calcium from dialysis is not enough. They also need calcium in the form of a drug. One commonly used form of calcium is calcium carbonate (usually taken in a preparation called Calcichew). Some renal units use another similar preparation called calcium acetate. Calcium tablets may need to be taken every day to look after the long-term health of the bones.

Although the main job of calcium in kidney patients is to reduce blood phosphate levels (see *below, point 2*), it also has the effect of raising blood calcium levels. Blood calcium levels are also raised by treatment with vitamin D (see *page 38, point 3*).

Treatment is most successful when blood calcium levels are driven to the upper end of normal. So the target blood calcium level for someone with kidney failure should be 2.4–2.5 mmol/l (given the normal range of 2.1–2.6 mmol/l). This target applies all the time for a peritoneal dialysis (PD) patient, and before dialysis for a patient on haemodialysis.

2. Lowering high phosphate levels. Dialysis removes some phosphate from the blood, but it does not do this very efficiently. Most patients therefore need further treatment to control the phosphate level.

To lower their blood phosphate levels, kidney patients are usually given tablets called phosphate binders. The most commonly used phosphate binder is calcium (see *above, point 1*). Aluminium hydroxide used to be given as a phosphate binder too, but is rarely used these days. Another drug called sevelamer (an alternative to calcium) is now being offered to some patients. To be effective, any type of phosphate binder needs to be taken just before food, and not together with iron tablets.

If the combination of dialysis and phosphate-binding tablets fails to control a patient's phosphate level, then it may be necessary for the patient to have more dialysis, or to eat fewer high-phosphate foods (see *Chapter 14, page 105*), or both of these.

Even with treatment, a kidney patient's blood phosphate level rarely returns to the normal level of 0.75–1.4 mmol/l. So the target blood phosphate level is not normal: it is a level of less than 1.8 mmol/l, and preferably less than 1.6 mmol/l. This target applies all the time for a PD patient, and before dialysis for a haemodialysis patient. This is difficult to achieve.

3. Raising low vitamin D levels. In a few patients, renal bone disease continues to be a problem even when the blood calcium and phosphate levels are brought under control. Treatment with a vitamin D preparation is then needed. The most commonly used type is called alfacalcidol.

Vitamin D treatment works in two ways: it provides the vitamin D that is lacking and it increases blood calcium levels (see a*bove, point 1*). PD patients receive vitamin D in the form of a tablet. Haemodialysis patients receive it either as tablet, or as an injection given during dialysis.

PARATHYROIDECTOMY

In most patients, correcting the blood levels of calcium, phosphate and vitamin D is enough to control renal bone disease, and cause PTH levels to fall.

In a few patients, however, this treatment plan is not sufficient, and blood PTH levels continue to rise – especially if the blood PTH level is over 100 pmol/l and not falling. When this happens, the blood calcium tends to rise to above normal (it is usually low in kidney failure). At this stage, the blood phosphate is usually very high. This combination of an extremely high PTH, a high calcium and a very high phosphate level cannot be treated by dialysis and tablets alone. An operation to remove the parathyroid glands will be needed. This operation is called a parathyroidectomy.

If an operation is not performed, the blood vessels (especially those that supply blood to the heart) can become 'furred up' with calcium, which can be very dangerous. Calcium may also be deposited in the eyes (making them red and itchy) or in the skin (which can cause parts of the skin to go black and die). A parathyroidectomy is a very effective operation. It returns blood calcium levels to normal, and can prevent these complications.

A parathyroidectomy operation takes 1–2 hours, and requires a hospital stay of 5–7 days after the operation. For the next few weeks, frequent blood calcium checks will be needed. This is because blood calcium can fall to a very low level after the operation. It is often necessary for patients to take high doses of calcium carbonate and/or vitamin D after a parathyroidectomy. These can usually be stopped at a later date.

TRANSPLANTS AND RENAL BONE DISEASE

If a patient receives a transplant and the new kidney works well, the blood levels of calcium, phosphate, vitamin D and PTH will usually return to normal, or near normal. Renal bone disease then improves, although it never really goes away completely.

If a transplanted kidney never functions properly, or if it starts to fail after working well, renal bone disease will become a problem. It is therefore important to pay attention to the calcium, phosphate and PTH levels even after a transplant.

BONE PAIN DUE TO DIALYSIS AMYLOIDOSIS

Renal bone disease is not the only cause of bone pain in patients with kidney failure. Bone pain can also be caused by a condition called dialysis amyloidosis.

This condition seems to develop 10 years or so after the start of kidney failure. It is caused by a poor removal by dialysis of a protein called amyloid. This causes a build-up of amyloid in the body, which continues even when a patient starts dialysis. After a time, amyloid is deposited in the joints all over the body, especially in the wrists and shoulders. This leads to joint and bone pain.

At present, there is no effective treatment for this condition in dialysis patients. Its progress is halted – to an extent – by transplantation.

KEY FACTS

1 Renal bone disease is an important complication of kidney failure.

2 Without treatment, renal bone disease can cause bone pain and fractures, and may also affect your heart.

3 All patients with kidney failure, whether they are predialysis, on dialysis or have transplant, have some degree of renal bone disease. Most will need treatment.

4 Renal bone disease is caused by low levels of calcium and vitamin D in the blood, and by high blood levels of phosphate.

5 A combination of tablets usually reverses these problems.

6 The best way of finding out how healthy your bones are in the long term, is to measure the level of parathyroid hormone (PTH) in your blood. The higher the PTH level, the worse your bones. A level of 10 pmol/l or below is usually satisfactory.

7 If the doctors cannot control your renal bone disease, you may need an operation called a parathyroidectomy to remove the parathyroid glands in your neck.

7 BLOOD TESTS AND OTHER TESTS

The information in this chapter will help people with kidney failure to understand the results of the tests they have.

INTRODUCTION

The majority of this chapter is concerned with blood tests, but other tests that patients may experience during the course of kidney failure will be explained in the later sections. Although the chapter is written mainly for patients on dialysis, the general principles described are also true for patients who have not yet started dialysis, or who have had a kidney transplant.

All patients with kidney failure have regular blood tests. Blood test results provide doctors and nurses with the information they need to treat their kidney patients as effectively as possible. Patients who learn to understand their own blood test results can find out a lot about what is going on inside their body. They can also assess for themselves how well their treatment is working.

THE 'FIGURES'

The term 'figures' is commonly used in hospitals to refer to the biochemistry blood test that most kidney patients have at the end of every clinic appointment. It is important to understand that every hospital will be using different measuring equipment and there will be some variation in what are considered 'normal' values throughout the UK. So don't assume you must have the same values as someone who attends a hospital 50 miles away. Also, hospitals occasionally change their 'normal' ranges. In addition, there may be differences in the normal ranges given for men and for women. The figures given in this chapter represent an average range, but do check what range is considered normal, for men and for women, at your hospital.

The biochemistry blood test is not really a single test. It includes measurements of a whole range of different substances in the blood. Most patients with kidney failure tend to focus on two of them: creatinine and potassium. This is a good choice, as they are probably the two most important tests. Both of them indicate how well dialysis is working.

However, looking at blood test results can give you a lot of information about your body. You (and the doctors) can gain information about the levels of minerals in your body, the acidity of your blood, the state of your bones, how well nourished you are, and how well your liver is working.

The dozen or so substances usually measured in a biochemistry blood test for kidney patients can be divided into two groups: dialysable and non-dialysable (i.e. those that are affected by dialysis, and those that are not).

TESTS FOR DIALYSABLE SUBSTANCES

The first group of substances measured in the biochemistry blood test for kidney patients are all dialysable. This means that they can pass from the blood into the dialysis solution, and vice versa. The direction in which a dialysable substance travels during dialysis depends on the amount of substance in the blood and in the dialysis solution. Substances always pass – by a process called diffusion – from a stronger to a weaker solution. (See *Chapter 8* for a more detailed description of this basic principle of dialysis.)

By putting more or less of different substances in the dialysis fluid, compared with the blood, it is possible to remove substances from the blood, or to add them to the body. The biochemistry test measures blood levels of several substances that may be removed from the body by dialysis – potassium, creatinine, urea and phosphate. It also measures the levels of some useful substances that are given to patients in the dialysis fluid – bicarbonate and calcium. Two other dialysable substances – sodium and glucose – are also measured, although the blood levels of these substances are not usually affected by dialysis.

1. Potassium. The chemical symbol for potassium is K. It is a dialysable mineral that is usually present in the blood. The normal level of potassium in the blood is 3.7–5.0 mmol/l (millimoles per litre of blood). Potassium helps the heart to function properly.

Patients with kidney failure tend to have too much potassium in the blood, although there are some patients who have too little. Either too much or too little potassium can be dangerous, eventually causing the heart to stop and the patient to die. Problems are especially likely if the blood potassium is more than 7.0 mmol/l, or less than 2.0 mmol/l.

There is no potassium in peritoneal dialysis (PD) fluid, and only a small amount (usually less than 2.0 mmol/l) in haemodialysis fluid. Because of the basic principle of dialysis (by which substances pass from a stronger to a weaker solution), potassium usually flows out of the blood into the dialysis fluid. Dialysis therefore normally removes potassium from the body.

Controlling the level of potassium in the blood can be quite difficult, especially in patients who are being treated by haemodialysis. Because of this, it may be necessary for some haemodialysis patients to restrict their intake of potassium-rich foods in between dialysis sessions. However, because PD is a continuous treatment, patients who are on PD will not usually find it quite so difficult to control their potassium levels (see also *Chapter 14, page 105*).

Despite the difficulties, a normal potassium level can usually be achieved.

2. Creatinine. Creatinine is a waste substance produced by the muscles whenever they are used. Like thousands of other body wastes, creatinine is carried around the body in the blood until it is normally filtered out by the kidneys and passed in the urine (see *page 1*).

Creatinine is not itself harmful to the body, but it is a very important 'marker', which provides a valuable guide to the levels of other, less easily measured substances in the blood. If there is a build-up of creatinine in the blood, there will also be a build-up of many other more harmful substances. The higher the creatinine level, the worse the kidney, dialysis or transplant function (see *Chapter 2* for more details).

The normal level of creatinine in the blood is 50–120 μmol/l (micromoles per litre of blood). There is no creatinine in dialysis fluid. Because creatinine is dialysable, it passes out of the blood, through the dialysis membrane (see *Chapter 8*) into the dialysis fluid.

Creatinine levels can never be normal when someone is on dialysis. This is because dialysis – whether PD or haemodialysis – can provide only about 5% of the function of two healthy kidneys.

For a patient of average size who is on PD, the target creatinine level is below 600 μmol/l. For a similar patient on haemodialysis, the target is below 600 μmol/l before dialysis, and below 250 μmol/l after dialysis. Larger, more muscular people produce more creatinine than smaller, less muscular people. Because of this, individual creatinine targets are adjusted to take account of body and muscle size. Provided this adjustment is made, the creatinine level is a very reliable guide to a patient's kidney (dialysis or transplant) function (see *Chapter 2* for more details).

3. Urea. Urea is a waste product of food. It is made in the liver and then travels in the blood to the kidneys, where it normally goes into the urine for removal from the body. Like creatinine, urea is a 'marker' for other, more harmful substances in the blood. A build-up of urea in the blood also indicates a build-up of many other substances. The higher the blood urea level, the worse the kidney (dialysis or transplant) function (see *Chapter 2* for more details).

The normal range for urea in the blood is 2.6–6.6 mmol/l. There is no urea in dialysis fluid. Again, because urea is dialysable, it will pass out of the blood into the dialysis fluid. Urea levels can never be normal when someone is on dialysis. Neither type of dialysis is good enough at getting rid of it. For patients on PD, the usual target level for urea is below 25 mmol/l. For haemodialysis patients, the usual target levels are below 25 mmol/l before dialysis and below 9 mmol/l after dialysis.

Blood urea levels provide a less reliable guide than blood creatinine levels to your kidney, dialysis or transplant function. This is because the amount of urea in your blood is also affected by what you eat and by how much fluid there is in your body. If you eat a lot, or if you are dehydrated, the level of urea in your blood will rise.

4. Phosphate. The normal level of phosphate in your blood is 0.75–1.4 mmol/l. In normal quantities, phosphate helps calcium to strengthen the bones.

Healthy kidneys help to keep the right amount of phosphate in your blood. But if you have kidney failure, the level of phosphate in your blood will rise. (See *Chapter 6* for more information about phosphate and the bones.)

Phosphate is a dialysable substance, and the aim is to reduce the amount of phosphate in the blood of people with kidney failure. This is the reason that there is no phosphate in dialysis fluid. Phosphate therefore passes from the patient's blood into the dialysis fluid (because of the basic principle of dialysis, by which substances pass from a stronger to a weaker solution).

The target phosphate level for dialysis patients is less than 1.8 mmol/l. It is not usually possible to achieve normal phosphate levels in dialysis patients. Dialysis is simply not good enough at removing phosphate from the blood. If dialysis does not keep blood phosphate at the target level, it may be necessary to take calcium carbonate tablets (as Calcichew, for example). Not only do these tablets give you calcium, they also reduce the level of phosphate in your blood by binding it together so that it can be passed out in faeces when you go to the toilet.

5. Bicarbonate. The normal level of bicarbonate in the blood is 22–29 mmol/l. If your blood bicarbonate is lower than this, it means there is too much acid in your blood. Acid is a waste product of food; like other wastes in the blood, it is normally removed by the kidneys. But if you have kidney failure, the level of acid in your blood goes up and the level of bicarbonate (the body's natural alkali) falls. If the levels of acid in your blood are not corrected sufficiently well over a period of time, this may contribute to malnutrition (loss of flesh weight, see *Chapter 14, page 104* for more information). Malnutrition is a common problem in dialysis patients.

The target level for bicarbonate is normal, preferably high-normal, say 26 mmol/l or over. For haemodialysis patients, this target applies after dialysis. It does not matter if the bicarbonate is always just above normal. It may even be a good thing for your nutrition.

In order to keep the acidity of the blood normal, dialysis fluid contains an alkali (a substance that is the opposite of an acid). In haemodialysis fluid, the alkali is either bicarbonate (at a concentration of 35 mmol/l) or acetate (at a concentration of 40 mmol/l). In PD fluid, the alkali is either bicarbonate (at a concentration of 40 mmol/l) or lactate, at a concentration of either 35 or 40 mmol/l. Both acetate and lactate are changed into bicarbonate inside the body.

The level of alkali in the dialysis fluid is higher than the level of alkali in the blood. Because alkali is dialysable, and because of the basic principle of dialysis, alkali passes from the dialysis fluid into the patient. In the blood, the alkali neutralises the acid and produces normal blood bicarbonate levels.

6. Calcium. Calcium is a mineral that strengthens the bones. One of the functions of the kidneys is to help to keep calcium in the bones. But if you have kidney failure, calcium will pass out of your bones. There is also a fall in the level of calcium in your blood. (See *Chapter 6* for more information about calcium and the bones.)

The normal level of calcium in the blood is 2.1–2.6 mmol/l. Calcium is a dialysable substance, which means that it can be given to kidney patients in the dialysis fluid.

If there is a higher concentration of calcium in the dialysis fluid than in the blood, calcium will pass into the blood during dialysis.

The level of calcium in dialysis fluid ranges from 2.0 to 3.5 mmol/l. Different doctors prefer different levels of calcium in the dialysis fluid – all have their advantages. Most dialysis fluids allow calcium to flow into the blood.

The target level for calcium is 2.4–2.5 mmol/l. This level, in the high-middle of the normal range, has been found to be better for kidney patients than a calcium level in the middle of the range.

If the dialysis fluid does not give you enough calcium to achieve the target level, it may be necessary for you to take calcium tablets (such as Calcichew, for example) or vitamin D tablets (usually as alfacalcidol) to help your body absorb calcium.

7.Sodium. Sodium is one of the minerals normally present in the blood. Its name is sometimes written as Na (pronounced 'N…a'), which is the chemical symbol for sodium. The normal level of sodium in the blood is 135–143 mmol/l. Sodium keeps water in the body, and helps to control the blood pressure. Some doctors think that keeping sodium levels low is important and recommend restricting the amount of salt you eat. In addition, we know that salty foods increase thirst, making it harder to limit the amount of fluid you drink.

Controlling the level of sodium in the blood is quite easy for people on dialysis. This is done by having a concentration of sodium in the dialysis fluid similar to that in the blood. (PD fluid contains 132 mmol/l of sodium; haemodialysis fluid contains 132–145 mmol/l.) Because the levels of sodium in the dialysis fluid and the blood are similar, dialysis does not have much effect on the blood sodium level and a normal level is usually achieved.

8. Glucose. The normal fasting level of glucose in the blood is 3.0–5.6 mmol/l. Glucose is a type of sugar, and it provides the body with energy. The amount of glucose in the blood is controlled by a substance called insulin, which is made in the pancreas (a gland in the upper abdomen). When someone has diabetes mellitus ('sugar diabetes'), either their pancreas does not make enough insulin, or their body is unable to use the insulin that is made. This means that their blood glucose level tends to be high.

Blood glucose levels are only usually a problem for those patients with kidney failure who also have diabetes. Blood glucose problems in these patients are due to the diabetes itself, rather than to the kidney failure that was caused by the diabetes.

For kidney patients who do not have diabetes, it is usually easy to achieve a normal blood glucose level. So blood glucose is not something that most dialysis patients have to worry about.

Although glucose is a dialysable substance, it does not do what people might expect it to do during dialysis. Firstly, for haemodialysis, the dialysis fluid contains an amount of glucose similar to that in the blood (about 5 mmol/l). As expected, given the basic principle of dialysis, very little glucose passes between the blood and the dialysis fluid.

Secondly, some of the dialysis fluid used for PD contains a lot of glucose. Even a weak bag will contain about 75.5 mmol/l (which is more than 10 times the normal blood level of glucose). In this case, it might be assumed that glucose would pour into the patient's body and cause problems, but in fact, the body deals with the glucose well because it enters the bloodstream slowly.

As the glucose enters the bloodstream, the pancreas produces insulin to bring the level of glucose in the blood back down to normal.

However, if a person has diabetes and can't use or make enough insulin, the blood glucose should keep going up. In fact it does not, usually. If a PD patient uses a lot of 'strong' bags (containing 3.86% glucose, compared with 1.36% in weak bags), the amount of glucose entering the blood may be too much for the pancreas to cope with. If a patient has diabetes, it may also upset diabetic control, making it necessary to inject more insulin, or to take more tablets. This extra glucose may make any patient (diabetic or not) put on body weight, usually as fat.

Given that glucose sometimes causes problems for PD patients, you may wonder if it is really necessary to include it in the dialysis fluid. In fact, the glucose in the PD fluid is there to perform one of the two major tasks of the kidney, i.e. to remove water from the body (ultrafiltration). Information about non-glucose solutions for PD is given in Chapter 9 (see *page* 61).

TESTS FOR NON-DIALYSABLE SUBSTANCES

The next group of blood tests to be looked at in this chapter are those which measure blood levels of various non-dialysable substances. Like the tests already described, these tests – measuring blood levels of albumin, and various substances such as bilirubin that show liver function – form part of the regular biochemistry test for patients with kidney failure.

Albumin. Albumin is a type of body protein. It is made in the liver and is present in the blood. The normal level of albumin in the blood is 34–48 g/l (grams per litre of blood).

The level of albumin in the blood is measured because of the information this provides about whether a patient is eating enough (especially enough protein). Kidney failure tends to reduce appetite. Also, during dialysis, some albumin and other proteins are lost into the dialysis fluid. Many kidney patients have a lower than normal blood albumin level. If a patient's blood albumin level is always low, malnutrition (loss of flesh weight, *see Chapter 14, page 104*) may have become a problem.

Unfortunately, the information obtained by measuring the blood albumin level is not very reliable. One difficulty is that the blood albumin decreases very quickly whenever a person is ill. This means that it is not possible to tell whether or not the malnutrition diagnosed by the test is really a long-term problem. Another problem with the test is that the blood albumin tends to fall whatever is wrong with a patient, no matter how well nourished they are. So, for example, if you have any infection anywhere in your body, your blood albumin level will fall. A further problem with this test is that, even if a fall in the blood albumin level is identified, there are no specific treatments to bring it back up again. The target level, for what it is worth, is normal.

LIVER FUNCTION TESTS

The results of a group of tests called liver function tests (LFTs) often appear at the bottom of biochemistry test results. Most doctors do not mention these, or brush over them, saying 'Oh, don't worry about them, they are just liver tests'. So why are they measured? The main reason is that biochemistry tests are generally done by a machine, which includes the liver tests automatically.

Having said that, patients with kidney failure can get liver problems. Haemodialysis, blood transfusions or a kidney transplant puts patients at increased risk of catching a viral infection (such as hepatitis B or hepatitis C) that can cause liver failure. Also, some of the drugs used to suppress the immune system after a kidney transplant can affect the liver. This is particularly true for azathioprine, ciclosporin and tacrolimus.

So here is a quick guide to common LFTs:

1. Bilirubin. This is the most important of the LFTs. (It is the liver function equivalent of the creatinine test.) Bilirubin is produced when worn-out red blood cells are broken down for removal from the body. The normal range of level for bilirubin in the blood is 4–25 mmol/l. Raised bilirubin levels show that the liver is not working properly. If the blood bilirubin goes above 50 µmol/l, the patient will develop jaundice (go yellow in colour).

2. Alanine transaminase. The normal range for alanine transaminase (ALT) in the blood is 5–50 iu/l (international units per litre). Raised levels indicate that the liver cells have been damaged by disease.

3. Alkaline phosphatase. The normal range for alkaline phosphatase (alk. phos.) in the blood is 30–120 iu/l. This test measures how well bile (a liquid made by the liver) drains from the liver. Bile contains the waste products from the liver. It is drained into the bowel, and leaves the body in the faeces. In patients with kidney failure, a high alk. phos. level can also indicate renal bone disease.

4. Gamma-glutamyltransferase. The normal range for gamma-glutamyltransferase (gammaGT) in the blood is 5–70 iu/l. Like alkaline phosphatase measurements, this test measures how well bile drains from the liver. GammaGT also rises if a patient drinks alcohol heavily over a number of years. A raised level can be an early sign of cirrhosis.

OTHER BLOOD TESTS

Kidney patients are also given a number of other blood tests in addition to the tests that make up their usual biochemistry test. The substances measured by these tests – haemoglobin (Hb), ferritin, cholesterol and parathyroid hormone – are all non-dialysable. Kidney patients have their Hb level measured each time they have a biochemistry blood test. Their blood levels of ferritin, cholesterol and parathyroid hormone are measured less often, usually every 3 months or so.

1. Haemoglobin. Most patients with some kidney failure have anaemia. Anaemia means that there is not enough of a substance called haemoglobin in the blood. Haemoglobin is important because it carries oxygen around the body. Every part of the body needs a regular supply of oxygen. (See *Chapter 5* for more information about anaemia in kidney patients.) The normal level of Hb is 11–17 g/dl (grams per decilitre of blood). If the Hb level is below 11.0 g/dl, the patient is said to be anaemic.

There is a very good treatment for anaemia called erythropoietin (EPO), which is given as an injection between one and three times per week. Dialysis patients who are not being treated with EPO may have an Hb of only 6–8 g/dl, which is very low. The aim of EPO treatment is to increase the Hb level to 11–12 g/dl. (See *Chapter 5* for more information on EPO.)

2. Ferritin. You need to have enough iron in your body if EPO (see *above*) to work well. The best guide to how much iron there is in the body is a blood test that measures the level of a substance called ferritin. The more iron there is in the body, the higher the level of ferritin in the blood and, generally speaking, the higher the levels the better.

For EPO to work, it is important to have a ferritin level of at least 200 µg/l (micrograms per litre of blood). The normal level of ferritin is 15–350 µg/l, but 200 µg/l is generally considered an an adequate level.

To keep the ferritin above 200 µg/l, many patients on EPO need to take iron tablets, or have regular iron injections. Some renal units now give iron injections to all patients with kidney failure, whether or not they are on EPO.

3. Cholesterol. Cholesterol is a form of fat present in the blood. High levels are thought to put people at risk of heart attacks and strokes. Current recommendations are to keep the level below 5 mmol/l of blood.

If the level of cholesterol in the blood is high, it can be reduced in some patients by going on a low-fat diet. However, many patients also need to take a tablet called a statin to control the levels.

4. Parathyroid hormone. Parathyroid hormone (PTH) is a hormone (a chemical messenger) that is made by four glands in the front of the neck. These glands are too small for you to see or feel them. If someone with kidney failure has low levels of calcium and/or high levels of phosphate for a long time, these glands grow and start producing too much PTH.

It is important to measure the level of PTH in the blood of people with kidney failure because of the information this test can provide about the bones. The amount of PTH in the blood is the best long-term guide to how much damage kidney failure has done to the bones. Blood levels of calcium and phosphate tell you

what is happening now; PTH also tells you what will happen in the future and, generally speaking, the higher the levels, the worse the bones.

Different renal units use different tests for measuring PTH, and different doctors have different views about PTH targets for kidney patients. The normal range is 1.1–4.2 pmol/l. Most doctors agree that a PTH level that is less than twice the upper limit of normal (i.e. less than 10 pmol/l) is generally considered to be satisfactory. As with phosphate levels, it is often hard to achieve normal PTH levels in people who have kidney failure. (See *Chapter 6* for more information about PTH and renal bone disease.)

OTHER TESTS

There are a number of other tests that patients are likely to experience at some time in the course of their life with kidney failure. The more common tests are described below. Some of these tests involve risks. You should always ask your doctor how a particular test will change your treatment and what the risks are before you agree to it. Not all tests that carry risk require a consent form (a CT scan doesn't, for example). So you can't even say, 'No consent form, no risk'.

For more information about tests while preparing for a transplant, see *Chapter 11, pages 82–3*.

FINDING OUT ABOUT KIDNEY FAILURE

1. Kidney biopsy. This test involves a hollow needle being used to remove a very small piece of the kidney, which can then be studied under a microscope. Biopsies are sometimes used to find out the cause of kidney failure. They are also used to check whether a transplanted kidney is being rejected.

If you are having a biopsy, you will be given a local anaesthetic to numb the area where the needle will be inserted. If a biopsy is being taken of your own

SUMMARY OF NORMAL AND TARGET BLOOD TEST RESULTS FOR PATIENTS ON DIALYSIS

Substance	Relevance	Normal level	Target level	Units
Dialysable substances				
Potassium	Heart health	3.7–5.0	normal	mmol/l
Creatinine	Toxin clearance	50–120	less than 600	μmol/l
Urea	Toxin clearance	2.6–6.6	less than 25	mmol/l
Phosphate	Bone health	0.75–1.4	less than 1.8	mmol/l
Bicarbonate	Acid balance	22–29	high–normal (26–29)	mmol/l
Calcium	Bone health	2.1–2.6	high–normal (2.4–2.5)	mmol/l
Sodium	Fluid balance	135–143	normal	mmol/l
Glucose (fasting)	Blood sugar	3.0–5.6	normal	mmol/l
Non-dialysable substances				
Albumin	Nutritional status	34–48	normal	g/l
Bilirubin	Liver function	4–25	normal	mmol/l
ALT	Liver function	5–50	normal	iu/l
Alk. phos.	Liver function	30–120	normal	iu/l
GammaGT	Liver function	5–70	normal	iu/l
Other (non-dialysable) substances				
Haemoglobin	Blood health	11–17	11–12	g/dl
Ferritin	Iron in blood	15–350	more than 200	μg/l
Cholesterol	Heart and brain health	3–6.0	less than 5	mmol/l
Parathyroid hormone	Bone health	1.1–4.2	less than 10	pmol/l

How do your test results compare? Although your hospital may use slightly different figures, they should be similar to those given here. If any of your figures do not seem to be on target, find out why.

kidneys, you will be asked to lie on your front. If the biopsy is being taken from a transplant kidney, however, you will need to lie on your back. After a transplant, several biopsies may be necessary over the first few weeks. After the biopsy, you will need to rest for 6–12 hours, but it is usually possible to go home the next day (or even later on the same day, in some units).

Kidney biopsies are not without risk. There is a 1 in 20 chance that not enough kidney tissue will have been taken, meaning that the procedure will need to be repeated. There is also a 1 in 20 chance of seeing blood in the urine after the biopsy. This usually clears up on its own but, in 1 case in 100, a blood transfusion is required. Occasionally, the bleeding is so severe that the kidney has to be removed in an operation. If you already have kidney failure, this can lead to the need for dialysis which can be permanent. There is also a 1 in 1000 chance of a biopsy causing death. So biopsies should only be carried out if there is a good chance they will provide the doctors with information that will change your treatment. It is always worth asking how the biopsy will affect your treatment before you agree to have one.

2. X-rays. Various types of X-ray are used to investigate kidney problems. X-rays may be taken of the kidneys, of the bladder – an **intravenous pyelogram (IVP)**, **intravenous urogram (IVU)** or **micturating cystourethrogram** – or of the blood vessels to the kidneys (**renal angiogram**, *see below*). These special X-ray tests usually require the use of radio-opaque dye (fluid which shows up on X-ray film), which may be injected into the bloodstream or flushed into the bladder during a cystoscopy (when a telescope is put into the bladder). There is also a small risk of worsening kidney function (as with renal angiograms), or even of causing death, with all of these techniques.

3. Renal angiogram. For this test, a special tube is passed into the femoral artery (a blood vessel in the groin). This plastic tube is fed up the artery, towards the kidney, and a special dye that shows up on X-rays is injected into it. The dye makes it possible to take X-ray pictures of the blood vessels of the kidney, which will show the doctors if there is anything blocking them.

A renal angiogram is a complex procedure which carries a degree of risk. Possible side effects include bruising in the groin (not uncommon) and pain. The X-ray dye can be toxic to the kidneys and may damage them. There is a 5–15% risk that a renal angiogram will make the kidney function worse. Although this is quite high, they normally recover. There is a 2% chance of the dye causing so much damage that the person will need dialysis earlier than expected, though in many cases once dialysis has been started the level of function at the time of the angiogram will be restored in time. A few patients will find they are on dialysis permanently however. In addition, a small number of people may be allergic to the dye. Complications following an angiogram can be fatal in around 1 in 1,000 cases, so (as for the renal biopsy) you should ask your doctor how the angiogram will change your treatment before you agree to have one.

4. Computed tomography (CT) scan. This is another special type of X-ray. It uses a machine to send X-rays around the area being looked at, in order to build up an image of the 'slice' of body being scanned. If you are having a CT scan, you will need to lie inside the machine for it to take place. You may also need to be injected with radio-opaque dye, and if you do – as with renal angiograms – there is a small risk it will make your kidney function worse. In very rare cases, the radio-opaque dye can even cause death.

5. Nuclear medicine scan. There are several types of nuclear medicine scan, which are becoming more popular as they are less likely to cause complications than X-rays, angiograms or CT scans. All nuclear medicine scans involve the injection of a small amount of a radio-active substance into the bloodstream. An 'isotope GFR' (glomerular filtration rate) is the most accurate way of measuring the kidney function – even more accurate than measuring creatinine level, eGFR or creatinine clearance. A 'DMSA scan' looks at the structure of the kidney (and is good for diagnosing reflux nephropathy, see page 6). A 'DTPA scan' is used for comparing the function of each kidney, i.e. to find out which one is working harder. (They should work equally hard.) A 'MAG-3 scan' is good at looking at both structure and function. The risks involved with having nuclear medicine scans are low.

6. MRI scan. MRI stands for magnetic resonance imaging – a scanning technique which uses magnetism, radio waves and a computer to produce high-quality pictures of the inside of the body. For an MRI scan, you will need to lie inside a large machine that sends signals to a computer. The computer then builds an image of the inside of your body. No X-rays are used. An MRI scan allows doctors to see good pictures of the inside of the kidney, which will help them to discover what is causing your problems. It can be a lot quicker than a CT scan.

7. Ultrasound scans. This is the same type of test as that used on pregnant women to check on the baby in the womb. It is also used to help discover the cause of kidney problems – either when kidney failure is first discovered, or if there appear to be problems after a transplant. It uses sound waves, so is completely safe.

Jelly is spread on the skin and an ultrasound probe moved over the abdomen and sides of the body, allowing the kidneys to be seen on the screen. Sometimes, the person carrying out the test may print photographs of certain images seen on the screen. The test is quick and painless for the patient, and tells the doctor if a kidney is shrunken, enlarged or even missing.

Ultrasound scans may be used to allow the doctor to locate the kidney before taking a biopsy.

TESTS FOR PEOPLE ON DIALYSIS

1. Adequacy test. Adequacy is a general term that refers to how well dialysis is working. Adequacy tests are basically **clearance tests**, as described in Chapter 2, pages 16–17.

2. Peritoneal equilibration test (PET). This is a test for patients who are being treated by peritoneal dialysis (see Chapter 9). The test measures how quickly waste products and fluid are removed from the blood during dialysis. It is an important test in determining the correct prescription for peritoneal dialysis. The test takes 4 hours, and involves taking samples of dialysis fluid and a blood test. Other similar tests include the **peritoneal function test (PFT)** when samples are taken from each bag used.

3. Residual renal function (RRF). When patients first start treatment, their own kidneys may still be working, but at a reduced level. The amount they are still working will vary from patient to patient and is known as 'residual renal function'. The longer a patient keeps their RRF, the healthier they will be. Over time, it is likely the RRF will decline, and in many patients, it eventually disappears altogether. As the RRF declines, the dialysis prescription should be adjusted to make up for the reduced function. A **creatinine clearance test**, which measures the amount of creatinine cleared by the kidneys and put into the urine (see Chapter 2, pages 16–17), is used to assess RRF.

KEY FACTS

1 The term 'figures' is used to refer to the biochemistry blood test that most kidney patients have at the end of every clinic appointment.

2 The biochemistry test is not a single blood test. It measures the levels of a dozen or so different substances in the blood. The results tell you and your doctor about the levels of minerals in your body, the acidity of your blood, and the state of your bones. It will also give information about how well nourished you are, and how well your kidneys are working.

3 The substances that are measured can be divided into two groups: dialysable and non-dialysable.

4 Dialysable substances can pass from the blood into the dialysis fluid and vice versa. Substances pass from a stronger to a weaker solution. This basic principle of dialysis determines the direction in which a substance travels during dialysis.

5 Potassium, creatinine, urea and phosphate are dialysable substances that are taken out of the body during dialysis.

6 Calcium and bicarbonate are dialysable substances that are usually put into the body during dialysis.

7 Non-dialysable substances measured by blood tests include albumin, various substances that measure liver function, haemoglobin, ferritin, cholesterol and parathyroid hormone.

8 If you have kidney failure, you should know the values of most of your blood tests all the time. What are they?

9 If you have kidney failure, you may need other tests to find out about the extent to which your kidneys have failed, tests to see how well dialysis is working for you, and tests to prepare you for a transplant.

10 Tests for finding out about kidney failure and dialysis include biopsies and angiograms, clearance tests and various types of imaging and X-ray. Ask about the risks of these tests before you agree to have one.

8 DIALYSIS – THE BASICS

This chapter describes what dialysis is, and explains how it works. The points covered apply to both peritoneal dialysis (PD) and haemodialysis.

INTRODUCTION

This is the first of six chapters which explain the treatment options available to people with kidney failure. There are basically two ways of treating kidney failure: dialysis (see also *Chapters 9 and 10*) and transplantation (see *Chapters 11, 12 and 13*). There is currently no cure. In other words, dialysis and/or a kidney transplant can replace some of the function of two kidneys (a transplant at most 60%; dialysis 5%) but does not get rid of the underlying problem. Kidney doctors will still consider that you have kidney failure, whether you are predialysis, on dialysis or have a kidney transplant.

WHAT IS DIALYSIS?

Dialysis is an artificial way of doing the work of the kidneys. It clears waste products from the blood, and it also removes excess water. The word 'dialysis' comes from a Greek word meaning 'to separate' – because dialysis separates the waste and water from the blood, and removes them from the body. It therefore performs the two main functions of the kidneys: toxin clearance (see *Chapter 2*) and maintaining fluid balance (see *Chapter 3*).

There are two different types of dialysis: PD (see *Chapter 9*), and haemodialysis (see *Chapter 10*).

HOW DOES DIALYSIS WORK?

Even though, at first sight, PD and haemodialysis may seem quite different, they work in similar ways:

- Waste products are cleared from the blood by a process called diffusion (see *page 52*).

- Excess water is removed from the blood by a process known as ultrafiltration (see *page 53*).

- Wastes and water pass into a special liquid – called the dialysis fluid or dialysate – for removal from the body.

- A thin layer of tissue or plastic, known as the dialysis membrane, keeps the dialysis fluid and blood apart.

THE ROLE OF THE DIALYSIS FLUID

Both of the key processes involved in dialysis – i.e. diffusion and ultrafiltration – depend on the use of a dialysis fluid. Body wastes and excess fluid can only pass from the blood if they have somewhere to go. The dialysis fluid provides the 'container' in which they are removed from the body. The dialysis solution is slightly different in each type of dialysis, but it does the same job.

The chemical content of the dialysis fluid affects the flow of substances between the blood and the dialysis fluid. During dialysis, body wastes and excess fluid pass from the blood into the dialysis fluid. Other substances, usually 'good' ones such as calcium, flow in the opposite direction, from the dialysis fluid into the blood.

THE DIALYSIS MEMBRANE

Dialysis solution is toxic to the body if it flows directly into the blood. It is important therefore to keep the dialysis fluid separate from the blood. This is done by using a dialysis membrane, which looks similar to a very thin piece of 'cling film'.

The dialysis membrane has thousands of tiny holes in it. These holes are big enough to let water, body wastes and various other substances through, yet small enough to keep the blood cells and proteins inside the blood vessels. So the dialysis membrane acts as a 'leaky barrier' between the blood and the dialysis fluid.

In haemodialysis, the membrane used is artificial, made from a type of plastic. The membrane, folded over many thousands of times, is situated in an artificial kidney (called a dialyser). Dialysis takes place outside the patient's body, in the artificial kidney.

In PD, a natural membrane inside the abdomen, called the peritoneum, is used. The peritoneum lines the inside wall of the abdomen, and covers all the abdominal organs (the stomach, bowels, liver, etc.). It is a thin layer of tissue, rather like a thin balloon in appearance and texture.

WASTE REMOVAL BY DIFFUSION

Diffusion is one of the key processes involved in dialysis. It is a process by which substances pass from a stronger to a weaker solution.

Diffusion works in the same way as a tea bag. When hot water is poured over a tea bag, the tea comes out of the bag and into the water. The surface of the teabag is like the dialysis membrane, as it lets tea drain out of the

The process of diffusion

1

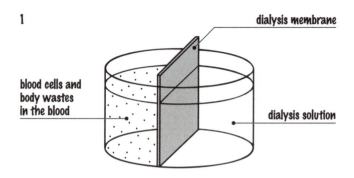

2

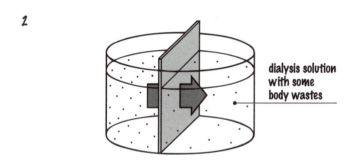

Blood cells are too big to pass through the dialysis membrane, but body wastes begin to diffuse (pass) into the dialysis solution

3

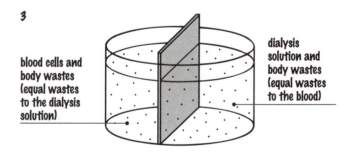

Diffusion is complete. Body wastes have diffused through the membrane, and now there are equal amounts of wastes in both the blood and the dialysis solution

tea leaves, but does not let the tea leaves out themselves. The tea mixes with the water until the tea is the same colour throughout the cup.

People with kidney failure have a lot of body wastes in their blood. If the blood is put next to a dialysis fluid that does not have any of these wastes in it, the wastes will pass from the blood into the dialysis fluid. So, if we want to remove unwanted substances (such as urea or creatinine) from the blood, we need a dialysis fluid that contains little or none of those substances.

As dialysis proceeds, there comes a point at which there are equal amount of wastes in the blood and in the dialysis fluid (as when the tea stops changing colour). The process of diffusion then stops, and no more wastes will move across. This is the basic principle underlying dialysis.

Diffusion also works the 'other way' round. If the amount of a substance is higher in the dialysis fluid than in the blood, then that substance will pass from the dialysis fluid into the blood. So if we want to add useful substances (such as calcium and bicarbonate) to the body via the blood, we use dialysis fluid that contains a lot of those substances.

FLUID REMOVAL BY ULTRAFILTRATION

Ultrafiltration – the other key process involved in dialysis – occurs at the same time as diffusion. It is the process by which excess fluid (mainly water) is drawn out of the blood during dialysis. Ultrafiltration happens in slightly different ways in haemodialysis and PD.

In haemodialysis, the water is 'sucked' from the blood by the kidney machine. The amount of water to be removed during a session of haemodialysis can be varied, from a lot to a little, depending on how the machine is set up.

In PD, a substance is put into the dialysis fluid which 'sucks' the water from the blood. The most commonly used substance is glucose (i.e. sugar). The way the

The process of ultrafiltration in PD

1

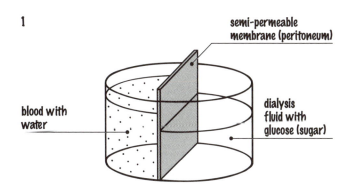

blood with water

semi-permeable membrane (peritoneum)

dialysis fluid with glucose (sugar)

2

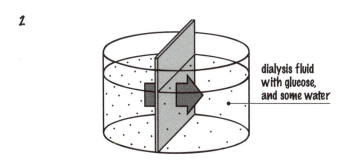

dialysis fluid with glucose, and some water

Blood cells are too big to pass through the semi-permeable membrane, but water in the blood is drawn into the dialysis fluid by the glucose

3

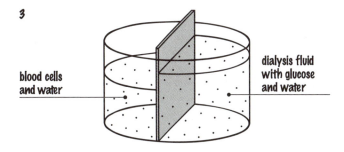

blood cells and water

dialysis fluid with glucose and water

Ultrafiltration is complete. Water has been drawn through the peritoneum by the glucose in the dialysis fluid. There is now extra water in the dialysis fluid, which needs to be changed

glucose sucks water from the blood is the same way as a tree draws water up from the ground to its highest leaves. It depends on a process called osmosis.

Osmosis occurs when a liquid from a weak solution (e.g. water in the blood) passes through a semi-permeable membrane (e.g. the dialysis membrane) into a stronger solution (e.g. one of glucose in the dialysis fluid). By this means, water is lost from the blood, and the glucose solution is diluted.

The amount of water drawn from the blood depends on the amount of sugar in the solution – the more sugar, the more water will be removed. Hence in PD, there are different strengths of dialysis bag – with 'strong' bags containing more sugar than 'weak' bags. The choice of bag depends on how much water needs to be removed from the patient's blood: a strong bag will remove more water than a weak bag.

PD OR HAEMODIALYSIS?

Both methods of dialysis are equally effective. Haemo-dialysis works much more quickly than PD, and so only has to be done in short sessions (taking 3–5 hours), two or three times a week. PD is a much gentler form of dialysis, and so needs to be performed every day.

Some doctors think it is better to start off with PD so, if the technique ever fails, the patient's veins are in a better state for haemodialysis at a later date.

In the UK, approximately 75% of the patients on dialysis are treated by haemodialysis, and the remaining 25% by PD. In fact, it is possible for most patients to have either type of treatment. Indeed, many patients will experience both haemodialysis and PD during the time they are living with kidney failure.

In most other developed countries, PD is not quite so common as it is in the UK. For example, only about 9% of patients in the USA are treated by PD. This difference could be due in part to the fact that doctors in some countries are paid according to how many patients they treat by the different types of dialysis. Doctors in these countries often receive more money for haemodialysis patients than they do for patients on PD.

KEY FACTS

1   Dialysis is the word used to describe the removal of body wastes and water from the blood.

2   There are two types of dialysis: haemodialysis and peritoneal dialysis (PD). Both work in a similar way.

3   There are two main processes involved in dialysis: diffusion and ultrafiltration. Diffusion removes the body wastes, and ultrafiltration removes the excess water.

4   In the UK, approximately 25% of patients on dialysis have PD, and the other 75% have haemodialysis.

5   Most patients can have either type of dialysis, and may well experience both at different times.

9 PERITONEAL DIALYSIS

This chapter concentrates on peritoneal dialysis (PD), one of the two types of dialysis that may be used to treat people with kidney failure.

INTRODUCTION

Peritoneal dialysis (PD) is one of the two types of dialysis that may be used to treat people with kidney failure. In PD, the process of dialysis (see *Chapter 8*) takes place inside the patient's body, using the peritoneum (the natural lining of the abdomen) as the dialysis membrane. PD has been available in the UK since the late 1970s. It has proved to be a highly successful alternative to the 'traditional' form of dialysis known as haemodialysis (see *Chapter 10*).

WHO CAN BE TREATED BY PD?

PD is a suitable treatment for most people with established renal failure (ERF). However, there are a couple of requirements:

1. A non-scarred abdomen. People who have had several major abdominal operations may not be able to have PD. This is because a scarred peritoneum may not be an effective dialysis membrane.

2. Commitment. PD requires a lot of commitment from kidney patients and their families. Kidney patients on PD are responsible for exchanging their own dialysis fluid (see *pages 57–8*). They perform these exchanges in their own homes. It is therefore a good treatment for people who are independent, or who want to be treated at home.

WHAT DOES PD DO?

PD (like haemodialysis) takes over some of the work that is normally done by the kidneys. It removes the waste products of food (toxin clearance, see *Chapter 2*), and removes excess water from the body (see *Chapter 3*). It can also be used to give people various substances that they are lacking, such as calcium or bicarbonate.

PD and haemodialysis are equivalent techniques in terms of the amount of dialysis they can deliver (about 5% of the function of two normal kidneys). Both relieve the symptoms of kidney failure, and both enable patients to go back to work.

HOW DOES PD WORK?

The basic principles of dialysis are the same for PD and haemodialysis. (These principles are explained in detail in *Chapter 8*.) Briefly, both types of dialysis use a special liquid (called the dialysis fluid, dialysis solution or dialysate) and a membrane (called the dialysis membrane) to do some of the work of the kidneys.

In PD, the dialysis membrane is the patient's own peritoneum (see below).

The dialysis fluid provides the 'container' in which waste products and excess water can be removed from the body. The dialysis membrane acts as a filter. It keeps the dialysis fluid and the blood separate from each other, but it allows certain substances and water to pass through it. During dialysis, substances pass from the blood into the dialysis fluid (and vice versa). They do this by a process called diffusion, by which substances pass from a stronger to a weaker solution (see page 52). At the same time, ultrafiltration occurs (see page 53). Excess water passes from the blood into the dialysis fluid by a process called osmosis, in which liquid in a weaker solution passes into a stronger one.

THE PERITONEUM

The essential difference between PD and haemodialysis is that, in PD, the dialysis process takes place inside the patient's abdomen, using a natural membrane – the peritoneum – as the dialysis membrane. It is from the peritoneum that PD (peritoneal dialysis) gets its name.

The peritoneum is a natural membrane that lines the inside of the abdominal wall and covers all the abdominal organs (the stomach, bowels, liver, etc.). It resembles a balloon in appearance and texture but has lots of extremely tiny holes in it. These holes allow the peritoneum to be used as a dialysis membrane. As blood flows through the blood vessels in the peritoneum, it flows past the holes. Although the holes are extremely tiny, water and toxins can easily pass through, but blood cells are too large. In this way, the peritoneum in PD works as a 'natural filter', performing the same function as the 'artificial filter' used in haemodialysis.

The peritoneum has two layers – one lining the inside of the abdominal wall, the other lining the abdominal organs. Between these two layers is a space. This space is called the peritoneal cavity. During PD, it is the

The position of the peritoneal cavity

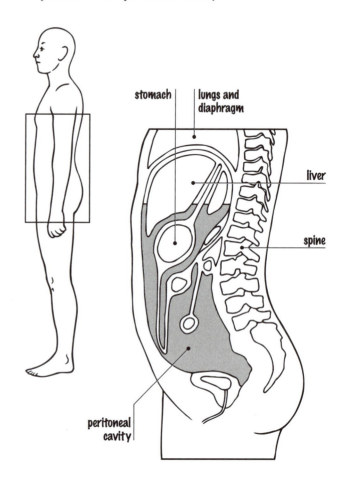

peritoneal cavity that is used as a reservoir for the dialysis fluid. Normally, the peritoneal cavity contains only about 100 ml of liquid. In fact, it can expand to hold up to 5 litres of liquid, as women who have been pregnant know.

HOW IS PD DONE?

PD needs to be done every day. It consists of the following three stages:

1. The peritoneal cavity is filled with 1.5–3 litres of dialysis fluid from a dialysis bag. (The amount varies, depending on a patient's individual needs and the type of dialysis fluid used.)

2. The dialysis fluid is left inside the peritoneum to allow dialysis to take place. (The length of time it is left there varies, from between 1 and 8 hours, depending on individual requirements, the time of day and the type of PD.)

3. The 'used' fluid, containing the water and toxins that the kidneys would normally have passed into the urine, is drained out of the body and discarded, usually down the toilet.

OPERATION TO INSERT A PD CATHETER

To receive PD, you will first need to have a small operation. During the operation (which is performed using either a local or a general anaesthetic), a plastic tube will be permanently inserted into your abdomen (*see diagram*). This tube is called a PD catheter. It is about 30 centimetres (12 inches) long and as wide as a pencil.

The PD catheter will be placed through your lower abdominal wall, into your peritoneal cavity. Half of the catheter lies inside your abdomen, and half lies outside. It will come out on the right or the left, under your navel (tummy button). The PD catheter acts as a permanent pathway into your peritoneal cavity from the outside world. Without it, you won't be able to perform PD, so it is important you look after it.

If all goes well, you will be allowed to go home 1 or 2 days after the operation. The catheter is 'left alone' for 7 days or more after the operation before it can be used for dialysis. This allows it to 'settle in' and gives the abdominal wound time to heal. PD catheter operations are not always successful – Only around 80% of those inserted end up being used reliably. So some patients

need two or more operations to get a PD catheter working. These may include a 'repositioning' or an 'omentectomy' (the removal of fat that has got in the way). However, this is still better than the results normally achieved for either fistulas or grafts in haemodialysis (see Chapter 10).

THE TRAINING

PD is performed by patients themselves, in their own homes. They therefore need proper training to perform their own dialysis. This training is usually given to patients two weeks after their PD catheter operation.

Before anyone is expected to carry out their own dialysis, they will be trained in all aspects of their care by specialist nurses. Most patients can become competent in the exchange technique in 3–14 days. Some hospitals train people as in-patients, others train them as

PD catheter – position inside the body

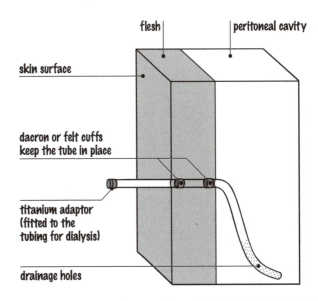

flesh

peritoneal cavity

skin surface

dacron or felt cuffs keep the tube in place

titanium adaptor (fitted to the tubing for dialysis)

drainage holes

Fluid exchanges in CAPD

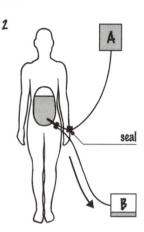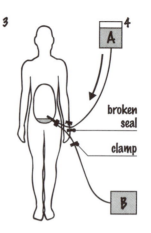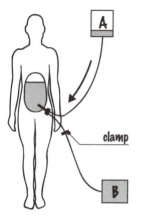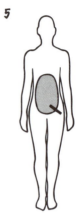

a peritoneal cavity
b catheter tube

1 Patient with used dialysis fluid ready to exchange

2 A Y-shaped tube is connected to the patient's PD catheter. At one end of the Y tubing is a bag full of fresh dialysis fluid (A). Used fluid is drained into the empty bag (B), which is at the other end of the Y tubing

3 When all the used fluid has drained into the drainage bag (B), the drainage tube is clamped to stop more fluid flowing down the tube. The seal is broken and fresh

fluid is then drained into the peritoneal cavity from bag A

4 Once all the fresh fluid is inside the patient, all the tubes are clamped and the bags are disconnected, leaving the patient free from the equipment until the next time a dialysis exchange is due

5 Patient with fresh dialysis fluid

out-patients, and some patients are trained at home. When patients first go home and have to do the exchanges by themselves, they may find it a bit daunting. However, within a few days or weeks most patients find they are doing dialysis by themselves with no problems.

METHODS OF FLUID EXCHANGE

The way that the dialysis fluid is exchanged depends on the type of PD.

There are two main types of PD, which differ only in the way that the dialysis fluid is exchanged. The two different types of PD are:

1. Continuous ambulatory peritoneal dialysis (CAPD). 'Continuous' means 'all the time' and 'ambulatory' means 'while you walk around'. In this form of PD, patients walk around with the dialysis fluid in their abdomen. At the end of each period of dialysis, they have to change the dialysis fluid themselves (see *above*).

2. Automated peritoneal dialysis (APD). 'Automated' means that a machine changes the dialysis fluid for the patient. The patient remains connected to the machine while dialysis is taking place, usually at night while they are asleep (see *below*).

FLUID EXCHANGES IN CAPD

If you are having CAPD, you will do your own fluid exchanges. This will involve draining 1.5–3 litres of dialysis fluid into your abdomen, leaving it there for 4–8 hours, and then draining it out. This is done 4 or 5 times a day – every day. It is as simple as that. With practice, an exchange of fluid can be done in about 30 minutes. Exchanges are simple to do and can be performed almost anywhere, and you can watch TV, read etc. while it is happening.

The dialysis fluid is kept in sealed plastic bags. The bags are connected and disconnected to the peritoneal catheter with a system of tubes and clamps. (How this is done is shown in the diagrams on *page 58*.) There are no 'set' times to carry out the exchanges. However, a 4-bag regime 'fits' into a typical day. For example, the first bag might be exchanged before breakfast, the second before lunch, the third before the evening meal, and the fourth before going to bed (leaving the fluid for the last exchange in through the night). It is easy for patients to adapt the timing of exchanges to their own individual needs. For example, if you want to go out for the day, you could delay your mid-day exchange, and do two 'quick bags' (say, 3 hours apart) after coming home. It may be safe to miss the occasional bag, but this is certainly not recommended on a regular basis. You should always check with your doctor or nurse before doing this.

FLUID EXCHANGES IN APD

APD uses a machine to do your dialysis fluid exchanges for you. Most people have their machine in the bedroom, where it does the exchanges while they are asleep. Some APD machines are only the size of a computer hard drive (see *above*) which make it possible for patients to do exchanges anywhere there is an electricity supply.

Most patients need to spend 7–10 hours attached to the machine every night. This enables the machine to

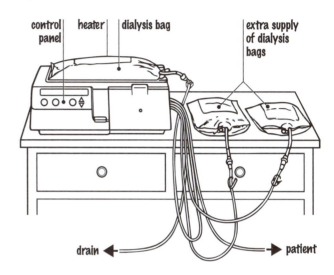

A portable APD machine

control panel | heater | dialysis bag | extra supply of dialysis bags

drain ← → patient

perform an average of six exchanges of 1.5–3 litres of dialysis fluid each night. The length of time that PD fluid is left in the abdomen before it is exchanged by the machine varies between about 1 and 3 hours. After spending the night on the machine, most people on APD keep fluid inside their peritoneum during the daytime without needing to exchange it.

A few patients can afford to miss one night's dialysis very occasionally. However, they should always check first with the doctor or nurse at the renal unit to see whether this is safe.

CAPD OR APD?

In most renal units in the UK, about 60% of the PD patients currently do CAPD, and 40% do APD. However, the number of patients doing APD is growing all the time. Different patients may be better suited to either CAPD or APD for a number of reasons:

1. How the peritoneum works. The main medical reason why a doctor may choose either CAPD or APD for a patient relates to the way the patient's peritoneum works during dialysis.

Some patients, called 'high transporters', have a peritoneum which works best with more frequent exchanges of dialysis fluid. High transporters are usually more suited to APD, because the machine is able to do rapid exchanges of dialysis fluid while they sleep.

Other patients, called 'low transporters', will get more dialysis if the fluid is left inside them for longer periods. Low transporters are generally better suited to CAPD. A test has been developed to find out whether patients are 'high' or 'low transporters'. This test is called a peritoneal equilibration test (see *page 49*), and is usually performed in hospital by a nurse. It takes 4 hours to complete, and involves doing just one CAPD exchange. The test measures how quickly the toxins move out of the patient's bloodstream and into the dialysis fluid. If the toxins move quickly, the patient is called a 'high transporter'. If the toxins move slowly, the patient is a 'low transporter'.

2. Patient size. APD can also be particularly good for patients who require a lot of dialysis – for example, large people, especially those who no longer pass urine. This is because the machine can do more fluid exchanges than patients are able to do themselves with CAPD. Also, as the patients are lying down, they may be more able to tolerate bigger volumes of dialysis fluid. (This is because there is less pressure on the abdomen when you are lying down.)

In these ways, APD can remove more waste toxins than CAPD. Even so, for some very large patients, APD during the night may not be enough. Such patients commonly need an additional CAPD exchange at tea-time.

3. Patients with a carer. APD is a possible treatment option for patients who need a carer to perform dialysis for them, such as the elderly, infirm or very young.

4. Employment reasons. Since APD exchanges are done during the night, this form of dialysis can be particularly suitable for patients who work or who are in full-time education.

BIGGER BAGS AND DIFFERENT TYPES OF PD FLUID

Whatever the type of PD (either CAPD or APD), the ability to remove toxins (i.e. clearance) can be raised by increasing either the volume of fluid used, or the number of exchanges, or both. A larger bag will remove more toxins (and a little more water) than a smaller bag. The dialysis needs of patients depend partly on their body size (see *Chapter 2*). Big people usually need 'big bags' (2.5 or 3 litres of dialysis fluid).

The ability of PD fluid to remove water (i.e. to do ultrafiltration) is affected by the amount of glucose (sugar) in the bag – the more glucose in the bag, the more water is removed. There are three different strengths: a 'strong' bag (3.86% glucose solution), a 'medium' bag (2.27% glucose) and a 'weak' bag (1.36% glucose). If you have too much water in your body (a condition called fluid overload, see *page 21*) you will be advised to use more strong or medium bags. These will remove more water than weak bags.

The strength of the bag is different from the size of the bag. A strong bag has more glucose in it than a weak bag, but it is no larger. Patients are advised to consider the weak bag as their 'standard' bag, and to try to use a minimum number of strong bags. This is because it has been noticed that using a lot of high glucose bags can damage the peritoneal membrane. The damage may mean that PD will not work effectively. In short, the less glucose you use, the longer you can have PD.

ALTERNATIVE DIALYSIS FLUIDS

There are a number of other dialysis fluids available:

1. Icodextrin. This fluid contains a glucose polymer (in which the glucose molecules are very large), rather than ordinary glucose. Because the molecules are so large, they cannot pass through the peritoneal membrane. Icodextrin may be recommended for PD patients who are diabetic or overweight. This is because the glucose polymer in Icodextrin is less likely than ordinary glucose to be absorbed into the body to cause problems with sugar balance or weight gain. Icodextrin has also been shown to benefit patients who have been on PD for a long time and whose peritoneums do not work very well for dialysis. It is also good for those exchanges which take place over a longer period, either the day-time exchange for people on APD or the night-time one for people on CAPD.

2. Amino acids. Some other dialysis fluids use amino acids rather than glucose. As amino acids are the building blocks of protein, and as some of the amino acids are absorbed into the blood, it is thought that these dialysis fluids might also act as food supplements. In addition, amino acid solutions do not contain any glucose, which makes them better at preserving the dialysis membrane. It also makes them particularly suitable for people with diabetes or people who are obese. It is claimed that dialysis fluids containing amino acids are useful for patients who do not eat well or who have malnutrition (*see Chapter 14* for information on diet).

3. Bicarbonate. A bicarbonate-based dialysis fluid has been developed to help patients who have problems regulating the level of acid in their bodies. The solution is very similar to that of the human body (it is 'biocompatible'), and is thought to preserve the patient's peritoneal membrane. This solution may also be good for people who experience pain when the fluid is drained in. Bicarbonate solutions are rapidly becoming the most commonly used basic solutions, and appear to be much better than lactate.

LIVING WITH PD

Once people develop ERF, they will have it for the rest of their lives. Without treatment – by PD, haemodialysis or a kidney transplant – people with ERF will die within a few weeks. With treatment, they will be able to do all or most of the things they did before they became ill. PD does affect a person's lifestyle – especially because of the need for daily dialysis – but the limitations are often less of a problem than many people might expect.

1. Flexibility. PD is a flexible treatment which can be performed almost anywhere. The dialysis supplies can be delivered to most parts of the world, and most APD machines are portable.

2. Responsibility and independence. People on PD usually do their own dialysis, in their own homes. This gives many PD patients a greater sense of responsibility and independence than is possible for the majority of haemodialysis patients (who receive their dialysis from nurses or dialysis technicians in a hospital).

3. Sport and exercise. Most types of sport and exercise are possible for people on PD. Even contact sports are possible (although not always recommended). If you are on PD and want to play sports such as rugby, judo and karate, you will be advised to wear a protective belt around your abdomen.

4. Swimming/baths/showers. Before a swim (or bath or shower), you will need to cover your PD catheter with a special plastic dressing, which you will be able to get either from your renal clinic or from your family doctor. After a swim (or bath or shower), you will need to clean the exit site of your catheter and, if possible, also do a fluid exchange.

5. Sexual activity. Most people stay sexually active while on PD. Some people may find it uncomfortable to have sex with the dialysis fluid in, but they can drain it out first and use a new bag afterwards. Patients on APD can have sex either before or after the dialysis starts. The connecting lead for the APD machine is very long and need not restrict you.

6. Stability. As PD takes place continually, all day and all night, people on PD generally feel fairly well most of the time. This is because their bodies do not have to put up with the rise and fall of toxins or fluid levels in the blood experienced by people who are on haemodialysis three times a week.

DELIVERY AND STORAGE OF SUPPLIES

PD is performed by patients themselves in their own homes. They therefore need to have supplies of fluid delivered to them and to be able to store these supplies in a convenient place. The bags of dialysis fluid come in boxes of two, four or five. So a month's supplies can be as many as 40 boxes. These can be stored in a cupboard under the stairs, a spare bedroom, the shed or even the garage.

Most people receive a delivery of supplies once a month, although patients with very small houses or flats may be able to arrange fortnightly deliveries. The people who deliver the supplies deliver to many other dialysis patients, and are specially recruited and trained to go into patients' homes. They will move the supplies to exactly where a patient wants them, and will even move boxes around so that fluid from previous deliveries gets used before the new stock.

POSSIBLE PROBLEMS WITH PD

PD is not always entirely trouble free. Patients may experience various psychological and physical problems:

1. Burnout or fatigue. PD requires commitment as it never goes away. PD patients have to do dialysis every day. Haemodialysis patients, on the other hand, do at least have some 'let up' from it – they do have 'days off'.

2. Body image problems. Some PD patients do not like the way PD affects their appearance. The abdomen may get stretched by PD, giving it a rounded appearance. Young people in particular may be very conscious of their body shape, especially if they are slim. Keeping fit and doing exercises to strengthen the abdominal muscles will help.

The PD catheter can also cause body image problems. PD patients have to come to terms with the fact that they now have a piece of plastic tubing permanently sticking out of their abdomen. Some people find this very difficult to cope with. They may also worry that the catheter might put off a sexual partner. (See *Chapter 15* for more information about the psychological aspects of kidney failure.)

3. Fluid overload. The amount of 'used' fluid that is drained out of the body after PD is about 1.5 litres per day more than the amount of fresh dialysis fluid that is put in. This extra fluid – in effect, the amount of fluid a person without kidney failure would get rid of in the form of urine – does not increase in quantity however much the patient drinks. This means that PD patients have to restrict their drinking to 1.5 litres a day in order to avoid problems due to fluid overload (see *Chapter 3* for details).

4. Discomfort. Some PD patients find that the dialysis fluid in their abdomen is uncomfortable. It may also lead to backache.

6. 'Wearing out'. The peritoneum does not actually 'wear out' but, in a small number of patients, it may in time cease to be effective as a dialysis membrane. Newer PD solutions, such as those that contain bicarbonate and no glucose, may help to preserve the membrane for longer.

POOR DRAINAGE

One of the most common problems with PD – especially among new PD patients – is poor drainage of the dialysis fluid. The PD catheter may become blocked with a substance called fibrin, which is a form of protein. It looks like tiny strands of cotton wool and is completely harmless. You may sometimes be able to clear the catheter simply by squeezing the tubing to dislodge the fibrin. Alternatively, a nurse will be able to clear the catheter by injecting water, saline (a salt solution) or a de-clotting agent, called heparin, down the catheter. This is a simple procedure and will not need an operation.

The most common reason for poor drainage is constipation. If a PD patient becomes constipated, the bowels press against the catheter and make the dialysis fluid drain very slowly. The fluid may also get trapped in pockets of bowel, preventing it from draining properly. So it is very important to avoid constipation, perhaps by taking regular laxatives.

Another reason for poor drainage might be that the catheter is in the wrong position. There is no single 'right' position for a PD catheter. As they are free to roam around the tummy, they can settle in almost any position and they may move into different positions from week to week. A 'good position', however, is one that enables the catheter to work well. Sometimes a displaced catheter will 'float' back into a good position naturally. If this does not happen, an operation may be required to move it.

LEAKS

In most PD patients, the 'seal' around the catheter exit site (where the catheter leaves the abdomen) works properly. PD fluid drains in and out of the abdomen through the tube without any leakage. Very occasionally, a leak may occur allowing the PD fluid to seep out around the catheter. However, this is extremely rare, apart from when dialysis has just been started. Fluid usually leaks only if the catheter has not been given time to heal before it is used.

If a leaking catheter is 'rested' (not used for dialysis) for 2–4 weeks, it will usually 'seal up' again, and become water-tight. Occasionally, however, a leak may recur even if the catheter is rested. It may then be necessary to have an operation to take out the leaking catheter. A new catheter, at a different site, is usually put in during the same operation.

In some men on PD, fluid leaks into the scrotum and causes swelling of the genitals. This is called a scrotal leak. If a scrotal leak occurs, PD will be stopped temporarily until the leak has healed.

HERNIAS

A hernia occurs when a wall of muscle weakens and lets an organ or tissue bulge through from inside. Hernias can cause difficulties for PD patients. If a patient has a hernia before the PD catheter is put in, it can become more of a problem afterwards. The daily draining of PD fluid into and out of the abdomen can cause the hernia to become bigger (and more painful).

If nothing is done, the bowel can become 'stuck' inside the hernia, thereby blocking the bowel. This will require an emergency operation. If an existing hernia is noticed by the surgeon during an operation to insert a PD catheter, it will be repaired during the same operation to stop it causing problems in the future.

If a hernia occurs at a later date, it should also be

repaired. This may require a 4–6 week period of haemo-dialysis while the operation heals.

PERITONITIS

Peritonitis is an infection of the peritoneum. It is usually caused by one of two types of bacteria (called *Staphylococcus epidermidis* and *Staphylococcus aureus*). In rare but serious cases, peritonitis in PD patients is caused by a fungus (usually a type called *Candida albicans*).

The most common reason why PD patients get peritonitis is that they touch the connection between the bag of fluid and the catheter. However, even if PD exchanges are scrupulously clean, infection can still enter the abdomen from the outside world through the catheter. PD patients can expect to get on average less than one attack of peritonitis every 2 years, so it is not that common. Indeed, some patients never get it. Patients on APD are slightly less likely to get peritonitis than those on CAPD, probably because fewer catheter connections are required.

A patient will know when they have peritonitis because the dialysis fluid that drains out will be cloudy. This fluid is normally 'see-through', and looks a bit like white wine. Patients sometimes – but not always – have abdominal pain and a fever as well. The treatment is simple and effective – usually one or more antibiotics given either as tablets or added to the fresh dialysis fluid. Patients are shown how to do this – i.e. they treat peritonitis themselves in their own homes.

A patient will not be offered a transplant if a kidney becomes available during an episode of peritonitis. This is because the drugs that are given after a transplant to prevent kidney rejection (see *Chapter 13*) may make the peritonitis worse. These drugs, which are called immuno-suppressant drugs, make it harder for the body's immune (defence) system to fight any type of invader (including germs as well as transplanted organs).

Occasionally, a patient may get several attacks of peritonitis in a row. The doctor may then decide that an operation to replace the PD catheter is needed straight away. The old catheter can be removed and replaced with a new one, at the same operation. Alternatively, the doctor may decide that it is better to remove the old catheter, and 'rest' the abdomen by not using it for PD for a period of 4–6 weeks. The catheter will then be replaced in a second operation. If this happens, the patient will usually need to have haemodialysis until PD is resumed.

If peritonitis is caused by a fungus such as *Candida*, it will be treated straight away – by an operation to remove the PD catheter. Drugs are not very effective against fungi, but the problem soon goes away if the catheter is removed. The catheter can still be replaced at a later date.

Patients who have had many bad attacks of peritonitis may find that PD is no longer suitable for them. They then have to change to haemodialysis as their long-term treatment.

EXIT SITE INFECTIONS

PD patients may also get another type of infection, called an exit site infection. This causes a red tender area around the exit site (the point where the PD catheter comes out through the skin). Also, when a person has this type of infection, squeezing around the exit site may produce some pus.

Some PD patients get exit site infections regularly, whereas others never get them. Keeping the catheter taped down to the skin will help reduce the risk of an exit site infection, especially when the catheter is new.

Exit site infections respond well to antibiotics, usually given either as tablets or creams. Sometimes, a single intravenous injection of an antibiotic called vancomycin is needed. There is usually no need to remove the PD catheter.

Occasionally, an exit site infection spreads down the catheter 'tunnel' (the route taken by the catheter through the abdominal wall). This type of infection is called a tunnel infection. Antibiotics are not always effective when someone has a tunnel infection. An operation to remove the catheter will then be necessary. It is usually possible to insert a new catheter at the same operation.

KEY FACTS

1 In peritoneal dialysis (PD), the process of dialysis takes place inside the patient's abdomen.

2 PD is suitable for most people with ERF.

3 Your own peritoneum (abdominal lining) acts as the dialysis membrane.

4 There are two types of PD: CAPD (a manual technique that you do) and APD (an automated technique that a machine does). In the UK, 60% of patients have CAPD, and 40% have APD.

5 Dialysis fluid from a bag is drained into the peritoneal cavity, left there until dialysis has taken place, and is then drained out.

6 If PD is the right choice for you, you will be trained to do the dialysis yourself, in your own home.

7 One advantage of PD is the independence it gives you. It enables you to take control of your own life and look after yourself at home.

8 You will need storage space in your home to accommodate bulky supplies of dialysis fluid.

9 Peritonitis is the main problem with PD. You will know you have peritonitis when your used dialysis fluid becomes cloudy.

10 HAEMODIALYSIS

This chapter describes haemodialysis, which is the traditional type of dialysis used to treat people with chronic kidney failure.

INTRODUCTION

Haemodialysis is the older of the two types of dialysis. This treatment became available in the 1960s, and since then has enabled large numbers of kidney patients to lead almost normal lives. The main difference between haemodialysis and the other type of dialysis – called peritoneal dialysis or PD (*see Chapter 9*) – is that in haemodialysis, the process of dialysis (*see Chapter 8*) takes place outside the body, in a machine.

WHO CAN BE TREATED BY HAEMODIALYSIS?

Almost all patients with established renal failure (ERF) can be treated by haemodialysis. The only real requirements are:

- It must be possible to gain good access to a patient's bloodstream (*see page 68*). (Access can be a particular problem for kidney patients who have diabetes, *see page 75*.)

- Patients must be able to withstand major changes in blood pressure and toxin levels. (Most people have no problems with this, but some patients with heart problems are unable to cope.)

WHAT DOES HAEMODIALYSIS DO?

Haemodialysis takes over some of the work that the kidneys can no longer manage when a person has kidney failure. Like PD, haemodialysis removes the waste products of food (toxin clearance, *see Chapter 2*) and removes excess water from the body (ultrafiltration, *see Chapter 3*). It can also be used to give people with kidney failure various substances that they may be short of, such as bicarbonate and calcium.

Either haemodialysis or PD can provide dialysis that is equivalent to about 5% of the work done by two healthy kidneys. This is enough to relieve most of the symptoms of kidney failure, and to enable people to do all, or most of, the things they could do before they became ill.

HOW DOES HAEMODIALYSIS WORK?

The basic principles of dialysis – which apply to both haemodialysis and PD – are explained in detail in *Chapter 8*. Briefly, both types of dialysis use a special liquid (called the dialysis fluid, dialysis solution or dialysate) and a membrane (called the dialysis membrane) to do some of the work of the kidneys.

In haemodialysis, the process of dialysis occurs in a machine. This machine is called a dialysis machine or kidney machine (*see top diagram, page 67*). Blood from the patient is pumped through the machine so that dialysis can take place. Dialysis fluid and water are also pumped through the machine.

The dialysis machine contains a special filtering unit called the dialyser or artificial kidney (*see bottom diagram, page 67*). The dialyser is a cylinder that contains thousands of very small hollow tubes. Each of the tubes is made from very thin plastic, which acts as the dialysis membrane. The patient's blood is pumped through the middle of the tubes. Meanwhile, the dialysis fluid is pumped around the outside of the tubes. The process of dialysis takes place through tiny holes in the tubes. Various substances and water can easily pass through the holes, but blood cells cannot.

During dialysis, body wastes (such as creatinine and urea) pass from the blood into the dialysis fluid. They do this by a process called diffusion, by which substances pass from a stronger to a weaker solution (see *page 52*). Meanwhile, other substances that are needed by the body (such as bicarbonate and calcium) can be supplied to them from the dialysis fluid. Again, it is diffusion (now working in the opposite direction) that makes this possible.

The second main function of the kidneys (and therefore of dialysis) is to remove water. The way that this is done in haemodialysis is not the same as in PD. (In PD, water is removed by a process called osmosis, see *page 54*). In haemodialysis, it is the action of the dialysis machine that removes the water. The machine applies a sucking pressure that draws water out of the blood and into the dialysis fluid. This process is known as ultrafiltration (see also *page 53*) or 'u...f...ing'. Instructions about the amount of water to be removed and the rate of ultrafiltration are entered into the machine at the start of each dialysis session.

DIFFERENT DIALYSERS AND MACHINES

There are many sorts of dialyser available, and different renal units tend to have their own preferences. Although the dialysers may look quite different from one another, the way in which they work is the same. The same applies to dialysis machines. Manufacturers opt for different colour schemes and shapes. Also, different machines display information in different ways, but they all tell much the same story.

How a dialysis (kidney) machine works

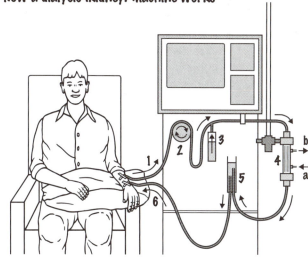

1 **Blood comes from the arm**

2 **Blood is pumped through the machine**

3 **Heparin (a drug to prevent clotting) is added to the blood**

4 **Blood enters the dialyser. Dialysis fluid with treated water (a) enters the dialyser, and wastes are taken away to a drain (b)**

5 **Blood passes through a bubble trap**

6 **Blood goes back to the arm**

A dialyser (artificial kidney)

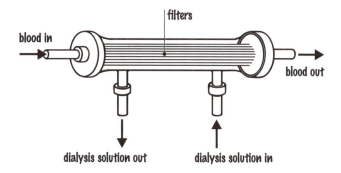

HOW IS HAEMODIALYSIS DONE?

To do haemodialysis, the patient must be connected to a dialysis machine. The machine may be in a hospital renal unit, in a satellite dialysis unit or, less commonly, in the patient's own home (see pages 72–3).

Haemodialysis is done by taking blood from the body and pumping it around a dialysis machine and through a dialyser. In the dialyser, toxins and excess water – which are the equivalent of the urine produced by healthy kidneys – pass from the blood into the dialysis fluid. The cleansed blood is then returned to the body at the same rate at which it is removed. Meanwhile, the 'used' dialysis fluid (full of toxins and extra water) is pumped out of the dialysis machine and down the drain.

Haemodialysis is usually done two or three times a week, for 3–5 hours each session. The exact length of the sessions will depend on the amount of waste that an individual patient produces; bigger people generally need longer dialysis sessions than smaller people. Longer sessions may also be needed by patients who do not pass any urine.

'ACCESS' TO THE BLOODSTREAM

The term 'access' soon becomes familiar to patients on haemodialysis. It refers to the method by which access is gained to the bloodstream, so that dialysis can take place.

During haemodialysis, large quantities of blood must be rapidly removed from the body, and (at the same time) just as rapidly returned to it. Therefore, in most cases, access has two 'sides'. One of these (called the 'arterial side') is used to take blood out of the patient's body. The other (called the 'venous side') is used to return blood to the patient after dialysis.

There are two main types of access:

- a fistula, which is formed from the patient's own blood vessels by joining a vein to an artery (see page 69); and

- a dialysis catheter, which is usually a double-barrelled plastic tube (see page 70).

FISTULAS

The usual form of access for haemodialysis is the arteriovenous fistula or AVF (often simply called a fistula). Fistulas are the preferred method of haemo-dialysis access because they are less likely to get infected and will generally last longer than the main alternative, a dialysis catheter (see page 70). However, some people are unable to have a fistula formed because they have very thin or delicate veins that are unsuitable for this.

Fistulas are made by a surgeon in a small operation, which may be performed under a general or a local anaesthetic. In this operation (see diagram, opposite), a vein (a blood vessel that carries blood back to the heart) is joined to an artery (a blood vessel that carries blood away from the heart). This can be done under the skin, usually at either the wrist or the elbow.

The blood pressure in arteries is always higher than the blood pressure in veins. When a fistula is formed, blood from the artery flows into the vein, and causes it to enlarge a little. Once the fistula has 'matured' (i.e. grown) it will be ready for dialysis. This usually takes about 6 weeks. If a patient is approaching the need for haemodialysis reasonably slowly, it will be possible to plan ahead and create the fistula at the best time. There will be a best time. If the fistula is made too early, it will have to wait to be used which is not ideal. But if it is too late, it will not be ready in time when the patient really does need dialysis. Most doctors would advise creating the fistula when the creatinine level is around 300–350 mol/l, or the eGFR is 15–20 mls/min. This is usually 6 months to a year before dialysis becomes necessary and gives time for the operation to be repeated if it is not successful first time.

Fistulas are not always successful. In an American research study, only 46% of fistulas were working after

A fistula

1 Normal vein

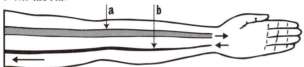

a Artery takes blood to the arm and hand
b Vein takes blood from the hand and arm

2 Vein diversion

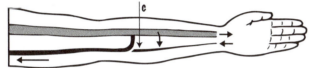

c A diversion of the vein is formed, linking it to the
artery in the forearm

3 Vein thickens

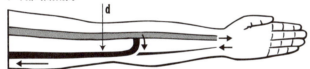

d The vein thickens beyond the link, and can now be used
as a fistula

one year, even with extra procedures being done on them to help them work. Brachial fistulas (fistulas at the elbow) may be more successful than radial fistulas (at the wrist) – i.e. more likely to develop into something that can be used for dialysis. However, although the success rate is lower for a radial fistula than for a brachial one, doctors will usually try a radial fistula first. This is because once a person has had a brachial fistula, they cannot then have a radial one. But if they have had a radial fistula first, and it ceases to work, it may still be possible for them to have a brachial fistula created.

Whenever a fistula is used for haemodialysis, a local anaesthetic may be applied to the skin and then two large needles are inserted into the fistula. These needles provide access to the bloodstream for dialysis, and are removed at the end of the session. Fistulas are a better form of access than catheters because they do not use any plastic, and so are less likely to become infected.

The creation of a fistula means some blood that would otherwise have gone to the hand (or arm) in the artery used for the fistula, instead bypasses the hand or arm and goes up the fistula. This does not normally cause any problems. However, occasionally, the hand or arm becomes cold and painful because of the blood that is 'stolen' from it by the fistula. This is called steal syndrome. Severe steal syndrome may mean that the fistula has to be 'tied off' – i.e. permanently blocked off – by a surgeon during another small operation.

Steal syndrome is more common in brachial (elbow) fistulas, which is a disadvantage of that type of fistula, even though the initial success rate is high.

When a fistula is touched, a buzzing sensation is felt. This is known as a bruit (pronounced 'broo-ee'). Patients with fistulas are advised to check for the buzz every day. They should do this gently as fistulas can be fragile.

If there is no buzz when a fistula is touched, this probably means that the fistula has become blocked by a blood clot. Often this occurs at night and is caused by accidentally sleeping on the fistula arm. If no buzz can be felt, it is important to contact the hospital as soon as possible as it may be possible to clear the clot and save the fistula.

HAVING 'DIFFICULT ACCESS'

Being told they have 'difficult access' is something no dialysis patient wants to hear. They know that whatever is about to happen, it will be painful (and may not work). The usual scenario is that a fistula stops working and a dialysis catheter becomes necessary. Even though these catheters are feared by some patients, they do have a role to play and can be life-saving. Knowing more about them may make them easier to accept. A dialysis catheter may be the best option from the start for some patients. Doctors can sometimes see that there are reasons why a fistula or graft may not work for certain patients and, if this is the case, a dialysis catheter may be the best option from the start.

DIALYSIS CATHETERS

A haemodialysis catheter is a plastic tube, usually with two separate barrels, one for removing blood from the body, and the other for returning it after dialysis. The catheter, which needs to be half in and half out of the body, is inserted during a short operation. This operation may be performed under either a general or a local anaesthetic. The catheter is inserted into a large vein either at the side of the neck, under the collar bone, or at the top of the leg next to the groin (see *diagram, right*). Names sometimes used for catheters in these different places are a 'jugular line' (at the side of the neck), a 'subclavian line' (under the collar bone), and a 'femoral line' (in the groin). It can be used for haemodialysis almost immediately after it is inserted.

Dialysis catheters may be temporary or semi-permanent. Temporary catheters are often used while patients are waiting for a fistula to be created. Other patients – particularly those with diabetes – have blood vessels that are not strong enough for a fistula, and will need a semi-permanent catheter for haemodialysis access.

Semi-permanent catheters are tunnelled deeper under the skin than temporary catheters. They also have small cuffs around them, just under the skin, to help keep them in place, and to help keep germs out of the body. Semi-permanent catheters also tend to be softer and more flexible than most temporary catheters. These tend to be used when a patient's fistula has stopped working.

After each dialysis session, saline (salt dissolved in water) is injected into the line to remove any blood. The

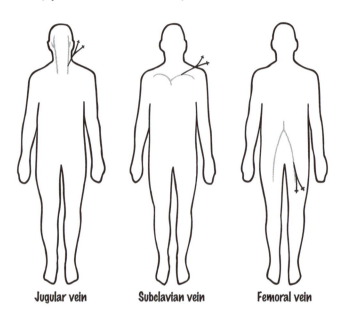

Entry positions for haemodialysis catheter lines

Jugular vein   Subclavian vein   Femoral vein

inside of the catheter is then filled with a drug called heparin. Heparin stops the formation of blood clots, which could block the catheter. This keeps the catheter clear of clots between dialysis sessions. Without access, patients who are treated by haemodialysis cannot dialyse. It is therefore very important that everyone – doctors, nurses and patients – all treat catheters with great care. Between dialysis sessions, patients are asked to keep their catheter clean and dry, and to ensure that it has a dressing on it at all times.

OTHER TYPES OF ACCESS

There are other types of access available, which are used when the two main types (double-barrelled catheters and fistulas) no longer work. This usually happens in patients with fragile blood vessels.

1. Grafts. A graft is a plastic connecting tube that joins an artery to a vein, inside the patient's arm or leg. (It is therefore different from a fistula, in which the patient's artery and vein are joined directly without a plastic connector.) The graft must be inserted by a surgeon during an operation. Grafts are made of a special self-sealing material (for example, Gortex) through which dialysis needles can be inserted. A graft can be used within days of being inserted. The operation is done much more frequently in the USA than the UK. In the USA, the success rate is probably better than for fistulas (59% working at one year, in contrast to 46% of fistulas according to the research mentioned on page 68). But the comparison is not entirely fair as different types of patient were chosen for the two techniques.

2. Single-barrelled catheters. It is sometimes necessary to use a single-barrelled catheter. This is inserted into the same sites that would have been used for a double-barrelled catheter. If a single-barrelled catheter is used, it is necessary to use single-needle dialysis principles (see below).

SINGLE-NEEDLE DIALYSIS

It is also possible to do haemodialysis using a single needle to remove and return the blood (rather than the two needles used for 'normal' dialysis). The single needle is inserted into a fistula or a graft. Alternatively, a single-barrelled catheter can be used. Single-needle dialysis is sometimes used for patients who have developing fistulas or grafts, or if a patient's fistula never enlarges properly. It is not nearly as effective as normal, two-needle dialysis.

HOW MUCH DIALYSIS IS NEEDED?

In most hospitals, it is the nurses in the renal unit who are responsible for working out how long kidney patients need to spend on the dialysis machine, and also what size of dialyser they will use. There are different sizes of dialyser – bigger ones remove more toxins than smaller ones (provide better clearance). Longer dialysis sessions will also remove more toxins.

As a rule, the bigger or more muscular the patient, the more dialysis they will need. In order to change the amount of dialysis that a patient receives, the nurse can choose to alter the size of the dialyser and/or the length of time that the patient spends on the machine.

The dialysis dose can be worked out simply by comparing the levels of wastes (such as urea or creatinine) in the patient's blood before and after dialysis (see *Chapter 2*), and making sure that there is a significant reduction. Some units still use this method, but it is now more common to use one of the newer methods of working out dialysis doses. The first of these uses a calculation called the urea reduction ratio (or URR); the other is a method called urea kinetic modelling. With each of these methods, dialysis target figures are the same whatever the size of the patient.

The urea reduction ratio is really just a more formal way of comparing urea levels in the blood before and after dialysis. As before, the patient's urea levels are measured in millimoles per litre (mmol/l) of blood, but now the measurements before and after dialysis are used to calculate a percentage reduction in blood urea. (For example, if the blood urea before dialysis was 30 mmol/l, and after dialysis it was 15 mmol/l, then the percentage reduction in urea during dialysis was 50%.) Such information allows adjustments to be made at future dialysis sessions in order to achieve the current urea reduction target of at least 65% per session.

Urea kinetic modelling also compares the levels of urea in the patient's blood before and after dialysis. However, this method also takes into account the size of the dialyser (called 'K'), the time the patient will need on the machine (called 't') and a number that reflects the patient's body weight (called 'V'). This produces a figure called the Kt/V (pronounced 'K…t…over V'). Because a patient's Kt/V figure refers to the amount of urea cleared from the body, the higher the number the better (see also *page 17*). A general recommendation is that Kt/V should be more than 1.2 for each dialysis session. However, as indicated on page 18, recent studies indicate that there is a point at which additional dialysis stops giving any benefit.

Some patients on haemodialysis believe that it is the amount of fluid that needs to be removed which determines the length of time that they must spend on the dialysis machine. This is wrong. The most important factor affecting the length of dialysis is the amount of toxins that need to be removed. However, if a patient has a lot of fluid to remove, they may need to spend extra time on the machine to achieve this.

HAEMODIALYSIS IN HOSPITAL

Most haemodialysis patients receive their treatment in a specially designed kidney unit within a hospital. This is called unit haemodialysis.

Patients attend the hospital two or three times a week to use one of the unit's dialysis machines. Unlike PD (see *Chapter 9*), in which patients have almost total responsibility for their dialysis, unit haemodialysis still tends to be done on behalf of the patient, by nurses, healthcare assistants and technicians. Patients therefore have very little responsibility for their dialysis sessions – other than turning up at the right time. This may suit some patients for various personal and medical reasons.

For other patients, however, the lack of control over their own treatment is not satisfactory. To help address this problem, many kidney units now encourage their more able patients to become involved in their own care. This may mean simply having patients check their own blood pressure before dialysis, but it may go as far as teaching patients to put themselves on to, and taking themselves off, the dialysis machine.

Visiting the hospital regularly for haemodialysis sessions does have its advantages. It helps patients to avoid the feelings of isolation that may occur when dialysis is done at home (either PD or home haemodialysis, see *below*). Unit dialysis gives patients with ERF frequent and regular access to medical and nursing expertise, education and support. It also gives them an opportunity to chat to other patients who are 'in the same boat'. Some frail elderly patients (especially those who live alone) can benefit from the social networks and company provided by having to come into hospital for haemodialysis. If their dialysis sessions are in the daytime, this may also be an opportunity for them to get a decent meal (which can be important as it is easy for people on dialysis to become undernourished).

SATELLITE HAEMODIALYSIS

Many hospitals now offer what is called satellite haemo-dialysis. This takes place away from the main hospital, in a 'satellite unit'. At the satellite unit, a small number of the hospital's healthier patients are treated by relatively few nurses. The patients generally do some of the dialysis preparation themselves. This allows patients to feel more in control of their treatment than is often possible in hospital-based units.

Satellite units can be more convenient for patients as they tend to be nearer to residential areas than many hospital buildings, making them more accessible by car or public transport. It may also be possible to arrange haemodialysis sessions after normal working hours.

HAEMODIALYSIS AT HOME

Some kidney patients can do haemodialysis in their own homes ('home haemodialysis'). The dialysis machines used today have many safety devices built into them, so it is usually quite safe to dialyse at home.

Whether or not a patient can have home haemo-dialysis depends partly on the hospital and partly on the patient. Some kidney units are more willing than others to provide home haemodialysis. Even if a unit is willing, the money must be available to supply the dialysis machine, to convert a room in the patient's home to be used for dialysis and to put in a special water supply.

To be considered for home dialysis, patients must:

- be quite fit, with no access problems;

- be able to learn to do dialysis, and be able to solve the various problems that might occur during a dialysis session; and

- have someone around to help every time they are on the machine.

As long as these conditions are met, home haemodialysis can be an ideal option for kidney patients who value their independence and who perhaps need to fit in haemodialysis around a busy work schedule. Also, bigger people (especially muscular men) can give themselves more dialysis than they could get in hospitals.

LIVING WITH HAEMODIALYSIS

The need to do haemodialysis regularly has an inevitable effect on lifestyle. Having to make frequent trips to the hospital can be an irritation, and may interfere with family or work life. Home haemodialysis may be less disruptive, but still involves a long-term regular commitment to the treatment by the patient and other members of the family.

If you are on haemodialysis, there may be practicalities that restrict your holiday choices. Holidays can sometimes be difficult to arrange because you will need to find a dialysis centre that is willing to treat you while you are away from home.

Some haemodialysis patients need a semi-permanent catheter to provide access, and they may feel unhappy about the effect this has on their appearance. However, the more usual form of access for haemodialysis is the fistula, which is much less visible. (See *Chapter 15* for more information about the psychological aspects of kidney failure.)

The patient and doctor may have different perceptions of what a 'good fistula' is. What the doctor sees as being 'an excellent, working fistula' may appear to the patient as 'a great, ugly bulbous thing that needs to be hidden'.

POSSIBLE PROBLEMS DURING HAEMODIALYSIS

Haemodialysis, like all medical procedures, is not without its problems.

1. Problems with adjustment. Most of the problems that occur with haemodialysis are related to the speed with which water is removed from the bloodstream during dialysis. Removing water from the bloodstream quickly is a bit like letting the air out of a balloon. When air is released from a balloon, the pressure inside it drops, and it becomes less rigid. In humans, when water is let out of the blood over a short period of time, the blood pressure falls making the patient feel faint.

2. Problems with timing. Haemodialysis is a more 'aggressive' form of dialysis than PD. In haemodialysis, all the dialysis is crammed into two or three sessions a week, each one lasting only 3–5 hours. In other words, the balloon is let down very quickly. The rapid changes in blood pressure (usually a fall), and in the blood levels of water and body wastes that occur during a haemodialysis session, can make some patients feel quite unwell, either during or after the session.

3. Symptoms caused by blood pressure changes. Fainting, vomiting, cramps, temporary loss of vision, chest pain, fatigue and irritability can all occur.

The best way to avoid problems caused by rapid physical changes during haemodialysis is for patients to stick to recommended fluid intake limits. For most haemodialysis patients, the recommended daily fluid intake is about 1 litre of fluid. (PD patients can usually have 1.5 litres.)

Some kidney units use a technique called 'sodium profiling' to prevent problems caused by the rapid removal of water. However, not all kidney doctors and nurses agree that this is useful. Although sodium profiling does help in the removal of fluid and does stop dizziness and cramps during dialysis, it may also make patients more thirsty after dialysis – and so more likely to need more fluid removing at the next dialysis session. For this reason, some people believe that sodium profiling creates a vicious circle of excessive drinking and fluid removal.

FLUID OVERLOAD AND HAEMODIALYSIS

Between dialysis sessions, haemodialysis patients sometimes develop the condition called fluid overload (see page 21). This causes excess fluid to collect first in the skin at the ankles and then elsewhere in the body, including the lungs.

Problems with fluid overload are usually due to drinking too much. However, the problem is not always the patient's fault. It can also occur when the person in charge of a dialysis session does not set the controls to take off enough fluid, or misjudges a patient's target weight.

If you think you may have fluid overload between dialysis sessions, you should contact the hospital at once. It may be necessary for you to have an extra dialysis session to remove the excess fluid. Constantly being fluid overloaded causes the blood pressure to rise. Like a balloon which contains too much air, the heart muscle stretches, and will eventually weaken.

You have the power to affect your own health. The best way to avoid the complications associated with fluid overload is to stick to the fluid restrictions your doctor has given you.

HYPERKALAEMIA (EXCESS POTASSIUM)

Another problem that may occur between haemo-dialysis sessions is hyperkalaemia. In this, there is too much potassium in the blood (see also Chapter 14). A raised level of potassium in the blood may cause the heart to flutter, and even stop. Hyperkalaemia can be very dangerous. It requires urgent medical treatment, and sometimes immediate dialysis. If you are on haemodialysis and hyperkalaemia is a problem for you, it is very likely that your doctor will advise you to be very careful about eating any food that is high in potassium.

PROBLEMS WITH ACCESS

There may also be problems with the different types of haemodialysis access.

As discussed above (pages 68–9) the usual type of haemodialysis access is a fistula, and if this works well haemodialysis will be technically easy. However, as was clear from the discussion of 'difficult access' (page 69) not all fistulas do work perfectly. Some never develop into a vein that is large enough for the blood flow to be adequate. Some function for months or even years, then suddenly stop working. In either case, a surgeon will then have to make a new fistula (or sometimes a graft) in another part of the body. Unfortunately, there are only a certain number of veins that are suitable to be used in this way. Anyone who needs haemodialysis for a large number of years may eventually run out of suitable veins.

To use a fistula (or graft), it is necessary to insert needles into it at the start of each dialysis session. Even with a local anaesthetic, some patients find this painful.

Because of the limited 'life' of fistulas, grafts and dialysis catheters, haemodialysis may eventually become impossible. This can be a particular problem for patients with diabetes mellitus (sugar diabetes).

Dialysis catheters may also cause problems. Some patients find it difficult to cope with their changed body image (see *Chapter 15*). Another problem is that dialysis catheters sometimes stop working because they have become blocked by a blood clot. If a catheter stops working, it will have to be replaced. Again, as for fistulas and grafts, there are only a certain number of veins suitable for plastic tubes. Dialysis catheters are more likely to become infected than either fistulas or grafts.

If a graft becomes infected, this can be very serious. It may be necessary to have another operation to remove the graft.

PROBLEMS ASSOCIATED WITH DIABETES

Over time, diabetes can cause a person's blood vessels to become very narrow. This can make it almost impossible to form a fistula in some patients. Inserting plastic tubes into the veins can also be very difficult. This is why some doctors recommend PD rather than haemodialysis for kidney patients with diabetes, especially when they first start dialysis.

There is also a fear that the drug heparin, which is normally given during haemodialysis to prevent blood clotting, can cause bleeding at the back of the eye (as well as other sites). Most people with diabetes and kidney failure are prone to this type of bleeding (a condition called diabetic retinopathy), by the time they need dialysis. Diabetic retinopathy can cause blindness. It may therefore be better to avoid having to use heparin.

However, not all doctors think that haemodialysis is inadvisable for this group of kidney patients. Some consider that haemodialysis is just as good as PD, does not worsen vision, and may indeed have some advantages for many people with diabetes.

BLEEDING

Haemodialysis patients may have problems with bleeding either during a dialysis session or, more commonly, after dialysis when the fistula needles are removed. Sometimes bleeding can result from using heparin during dialysis. So most centres now try to use as little heparin as possible, and some people have heparin-free dialysis. To try to stop the bleeding after dialysis, it is common for the heparin to be turned off at least 1 hour before the end of the dialysis session.

INFECTIONS

There is always a risk that a patient will pick up an infection during a dialysis session. Germs may enter the patient's blood either from the haemodialysis access or from the lines of the machine. During sessions of dialysis, fevers often become worse and there may be rigors (shivering attacks).

Infections can usually be treated with antibiotics, but it is better to avoid getting an infection in the first place. This can be achieved by strict attention to hygiene. Care is needed both with personal hygiene and when the dialysis machine and access lines are set up. Fistulas are much less likely to get infected than dialysis catheters.

Patients may sometimes develop an infection where the haemodialysis catheter comes out from under the skin. This is called an exit site infection, and causes the area around the catheter to become sore and inflamed. Most exit site infections respond well to antibiotics.

The inside of the catheter can also become infected. This is called a line infection, and can make you very unwell, causing fever and rigors. If you develop a line infection, your catheter may be removed and replaced after the fever has settled. But if you don't have many other possible sites for access, it may be left in until you have had 3 or more infections. A very bad infection will mean it has to be taken out immediately even if there are few other options. Temporary catheters are more likely to become infected than semi-permanent ones, and for this reason temporary catheters should be replaced after about 3 weeks of use even if they are not obviously infected. This helps to prevent line infections.

TAKING CONTROL OF YOUR LIFE ON HAEMODIALYSIS

Life on haemodialysis can feel restricted. However, people who have haemodialysis will generally feel better and able to do more if they look after themselves. Making sure you don't get fluid overloaded between dialysis sessions will certainly help your health. It is also important to talk regularly to the nurses and dietitians, to see whether your blood test results are OK. You may need to restrict some things that you eat, e.g. if they contain salt or potassium. If you take an interest in your diet and ask for advice, you will feel more in control and you will probably be healthier.

KEY FACTS

1 In haemodialysis, the process of dialysis takes place inside a machine.

2 Haemodialysis is suitable for most people with kidney failure.

3 In a haemodialysis session, blood is taken from the body, pumped into the dialysis machine, cleaned by an artificial kidney (dialyser), and pumped back into the body.

4 Haemodialysis is usually done 2 or 3 times a week, each session lasting 3–5 hours.

5 If you are going to do haemodialysis, you will need direct access to your bloodstream. The usual types of access are a fistula (made by joining a vein to an artery) or a dialysis catheter.

6 Most patients have haemodialysis in hospital, but (depending on where you live) you may be able to have it in a satellite dialysis unit or at home.

7 Some people feel sick or dizzy during a haemodialysis session. This is usually due to the rapid removal of water and toxins, which results in a rapid drop in blood pressure.

8 If you are on haemodialysis, you will need to control the amount of fluid you drink more strictly than if you were on PD.

9 Fistulas, grafts and dialysis catheters all have a limited life. In practice, this means that haemodialysis may eventually become impossible for some people.

11 TRANSPLANTATION

This is the first of three chapters that provide information about kidney transplants. It covers the issues and the various procedures that are necessary before a patient can have the operation.

INTRODUCTION

A successful kidney transplant is a more effective treatment for kidney failure than either peritoneal dialysis (see *Chapter 9*) or haemodialysis (see *Chapter 10*). This is because a well-functioning transplanted kidney can do all the jobs of the old kidney, whereas dialysis only really does a couple of these jobs. However, not all patients are suitable for transplantation, and not all suitable patients are suitable all the time.

Also, before a transplant can take place, it is necessary to find an appropriate donor kidney, which may not be easy.

THE BENEFITS

A kidney transplant can deliver the best quality of life to people with ERF. There is no doubt that for the right patient at the right time, a transplant is the best treatment option. A 'good' transplant provides about 60% of the function of two normal kidneys (compared with only about 5% from either type of dialysis). Then the blood creatinine level will be under 200 µmol/l (i.e. a stable transplant patient with a well-functioning kidney will still have chronic kidney failure at Stages 2–3).

The most obvious advantage of a transplant to people with kidney failure is freedom from dialysis. If a transplant works well, dialysis becomes a thing of the past. There are also no particular fluid or dietary restrictions after a transplant. Erythropoietin and calcium tablets, such as Calcichew, can usually be stopped. Most people who have had a transplant feel better and have more energy than they did on dialysis. They are better able to cope with a job, and many find their sex lives improve. Women are more likely to get pregnant and have a healthy baby.

WHO CAN HAVE A TRANSPLANT?

Up to 40% of patients with kidney failure are suitable for a transplant, provided a suitable donor kidney can be found (see *page 79*). Patients who will probably not be considered suitable include anyone with serious heart or lung disease, or with many types of cancer.

Most kidney units do not have an age limit for kidney transplantation. Patients are considered on merit (i.e. their suitability for a transplant) rather than age. However, having said that, most units would think very seriously before transplanting a patient over 70 years old.

Doctors do not believe that transplanting an older patient 'wastes' a kidney that a younger person would get 'more benefit' from. The main reason for limiting transplants among older patients is that they often do not tolerate the operation very well. Also, the drugs that are needed after a transplant (see *page 98*) are often too strong for older patients.

NEW KIDNEYS AND OLD DISEASES

Patients who are having kidney transplants sometimes worry that the original cause of their kidney failure might make the new kidney fail too, but this would be very unusual for most people. An exception, however, is where the original kidneys failed because the patient had a condition called focal and segmental glomulerosclerosis (FSGS). This is a type of glomerulonephritis, and it comes back in around 20% of patients who have had it before. Patients who have lost one kidney due to recurrent FSGS have a 50% chance of losing another one.

There are a few other types of glomerulonephritis and related conditions that may also come back and affect the transplanted kidney. These include mesangiocapillary glomerulonephritis (variable, depending on type), Goodpasture's disease (25%), haemolytic uraemic syndrome (less than 25%), membranous nephropathy (less than 25%), IgA nephropathy (10%), Henoch-Schönlein purpura (10%), and lupus nephritis (1%). But these conditions, if they do recur, do not necessarily lead to loss of the kidney. However, if FSGS or one of these other conditions were to recur in two consecutive kidneys (causing their failure) doctors would be unlikely to recommend a third transplant.

Patients who are affected by any of these conditions, should ask their doctor about the likelihood of the original disease recurring, and damaging a kidney transplant.

DO YOU HAVE TO BE ON DIALYSIS FIRST?

Most kidney units will not put patients onto the national waiting list for a transplant kidney (see page 82) until they are stable on dialysis. However, a few units will put patients onto the list before this point. This is usually done when the blood creatinine is about 400 µmol/l (micromoles per litre of blood) and the eGFR

10–15 mls/minute – i.e. about 6 months before dialysis will be needed. Also, if someone has a transplant that is failing, they may be put onto the list at this same point, and given a new kidney before they have to go back on dialysis.

The national waiting list is for what is known as a cadaveric transplant (see page 80). This type of transplant uses a kidney that has been removed from someone who has died; 72% of the kidneys transplanted in the UK come from this source. The remaining 28% are what are known as living related transplants or LRTs, and living unrelated transplants or LURTs (see page 89). For some patients, the possibility of obtaining a transplant kidney from a living donor will be the best chance of having a transplant operation before dialysis is needed.

Given that it is possible for people with kidney failure to be given a transplant before they need dialysis, you may wonder why all hospitals don't do this. The reason is that most doctors think that because there is such a shortage of kidneys for transplantation, it is better if patients all around the UK start waiting for a kidney at an equivalent time point, i.e. when they start dialysis. This makes it fair for everyone.

However, some kidney units are undoubtedly better organised in terms of transplantation than others. So some units do carry out more transplants before dialysis. Some units also make more effort to obtain kidneys than others and do more transplants, and some units are keener on living transplants than others. For all these reasons, patients in some units may wait less time for a transplant; and be more likely to have a transplant before they need dialysis, than is usual in other units.

You have a right to ask the doctors, nurses or managers about the performance of your unit. You may want to ask them how many transplant operations they do, and how long (on average) these transplanted kidneys last. How many of the transplants they carry out are of kidneys from living donors? Can you have a transplant from a living donor before you need to go onto dialysis? You have a right to know the answers to these questions, and the data are all on the UK Transplant website (see *page 162* for address). You will find that performance does vary quite considerably around the UK.

FINDING A SUITABLE KIDNEY

For a kidney transplant to be successful, it is better that the tissues of the new kidney are fairly similar (i.e. 'matched') to the patient's original kidney. If the new kidney is not a good enough match, the patient's immune system (natural defence system) will be more likely to attack and reject it. (See *page 96* for a description of the rejection process.)

Before a suitable kidney can be looked for, it is necessary for patients to have a number of tests. The most important of these are to find out the patient's blood group (see *below*) and tissue type (see *page 80*). The results will then be checked against the results of similar tests carried out either on an available kidney, or on a relative or other person who is considering donating one of their kidneys to the patient.

MATCHING THE BLOOD GROUP

The blood group is an inherited characteristic of red blood cells. It stays the same throughout your life. There are four main blood groups. These groups are called A, B, AB and O. Group O is the most common, followed by group A – except in Asian patients, in whom group B is the most common.

The blood group that you belong to depends on whether or not you have certain substances called antigens (types of protein) in your body. Two different antigens – called A and B – determine a person's blood group. If you have these antigens, they will be on the outer surface of all your cells, not just on your blood

cells. If you have only antigen A, your blood group is A. If you have only antigen B, your blood group is B. If you have both antigen A and antigen B, your blood group is AB. If you have neither of these antigens, your blood group is O.

The function of the blood group antigens is not known exactly. They may act as a 'friendly face' for the cells, so the rest of the body can recognise the cells as their own, and leave them alone. A person's immune system will attack any cells that have a foreign antigen. This means a patient can only be given a transplant kidney if the patient's and donor's blood groups are matched as follows:

Patient	Donor
Group O	Group O
Group A	Group A or group O
Group B	Group B or group O
Group AB	Any group (O, A, B, or AB)

MATCHING THE TISSUE TYPE

The principle of matching for tissue type is similar to that for matching for blood group. Again, the patient and the donor kidney or potential donor are matched using a blood test. The tissue typing test shows a person's genetic make-up (a type of 'genetic fingerprint').

The tissue type is an inherited set of characteristics (antigens) on the surface of most cells. It stays the same throughout your life. You have only one tissue type (just as you only have one blood group), but your tissue type is made up of six different tissue type characteristics.

There are three main sorts of tissue type characteristic, called A, B and DR. Everyone has two of each (one from each parent) – making six in all. Just to make it more complicated, there are many different types of A, B and DR characteristic. In fact there are 20 or more different versions of each A, B and DR characteristic. This means that there are hundreds of different possible tissue types. So, for example, a tissue type could be A1/A2, B7/B8, DR2/DR3.

As there are so many possible tissue types, matching tissue types is a little more complicated than matching blood groups. However, basically the more of these that are the same for both patient and donor kidney, the better will be the chances that the transplant kidney will work.

Given the large number of tissue type possibilities, it is very unusual to get an exact match (known as a '6 out of 6 match' or 'full-house match') between a patient and donor. Most units will offer a transplant if the patient and donor have three or more of the six tissue type characteristics in common, and there is at least one DR match. In terms of tissue typing, it is more important that the DR characteristics are matched than the A or B types. So, for example, a transplant might be offered in the following situation:

Patient:	A1/A2	B7/B8	DR2/DR3
Donor:	A1/A3	B7/B12	DR2/DR7

As the A1, B7 and DR2 characteristics are the same in this example. It would be called a '3 out of 6 match, including one DR match'.

The more characteristics that match the better. So a '6 out of 6 match' is better than a '3 out of 6 match'. The better the match, the more likely it is that the body will accept the kidney 'as its own', and not try to reject it.

Unfortunately, it cannot be guaranteed that even a '6 out of 6' match will not be rejected. This is because the blood group and tissue type are not the only cell surface characteristics that are important. However, these other important characteristics have not yet all been identified. Tissue-type matching is less important for transplants from living donors where a 1 out of 6 match may be satisfactory (see page 85).

TESTING FOR VIRUSES

Before a patient can be put forward for a transplant, they will have to be tested for various viruses. These include HIV (the virus that causes AIDS), hepatitis B, hepatitis C and cytomegalovirus (CMV). It is important to test for these viruses because they may be dormant ('sleeping', causing no symptoms) in a patient's body. After the transplant, they may be 'woken up' and cause illness. This is especially true of CMV.

Patients who refuse to have any of these tests, such as the HIV test, will not be able to have a transplant. If a patient has one of the viruses, it does not mean that they will not get a transplant, it just means the doctors will have to be more careful.

OTHER TESTS FOR TRANSPLANT SUITABILITY

Other tests are also necessary before a patient can have a transplant. These include an electrocardiogram (ECG, an electric recording of the heart beat), a chest X-ray, and sometimes an echocardiogram (ECHO, a sound-wave picture of the heart) and an 'exercise test' (a test in which the patient has to walk on a moving walkway, to test their fitness, and stress the heart). Some kidney units also insist that kidney patients who are diabetic also have a cardiac catheter test (a special X-ray picture of the heart). This cardiac test has some risk, causing death in 1 in 1,000 patients.

If results of all these tests are satisfactory, the patient can then be put on the national waiting list (see page 82) for a cadaveric transplant, or considered for a possible transplant from a living donor.

CADAVERIC TRANSPLANTS (AND HOW LONG THEY LAST)

The term 'cadaveric transplant' is used to describe a transplant kidney that has been removed from someone who has died. In 2004, 72% of transplant kidneys in the

UK came from this source, and current follow-up studies indicate that 88% (about 9 out of 10) are working after the first year (see also *page 86*).

But what do all these percentages and fractions mean for you? In other words, how long will *your* kidney last? Well, it's difficult to say, but on average, a cadaveric transplant will last about 7 years. But yours may last 5 minutes or 20 years, or it may not work at all. But the average is 7 years. Doctors have still not been able to make cadaveric kidney transplants last a very long time.

WHERE DO CADAVERIC KIDNEYS COME FROM?

Most of these donors have been killed in car accidents or died from a stroke, and have been on a life support machine (ventilator) in an intensive care unit. The ventilator is breathing for them. Their kidneys can be removed after the person has been diagnosed 'brain dead'. This means the part of the brain called the brainstem, which controls breathing, has permanently stopped working, and the person is legally certified as dead. The doctors then record this in the medical notes.

Once brainstem death is diagnosed, this is irreversible, and the person's ability to breathe for themselves will not return. An individual who is brainstem dead cannot remain on a life support machine indefinitely, as their heart will stop relatively soon.

If the person on the life support machine is not going to be a donor, their machine would be switched off at this point. If they are going to be a donor, their kidneys for donation are usually removed immediately after the donor's heart has stopped beating, which occurs shortly after the life support machine has been switched off. For this reason, these donors are sometimes called 'heart-beating donors'.

NON-HEART-BEATING AND LIVING DONORS

Because of the shortage of donors, some kidney units are obtaining transplant kidneys from people who have died up to 30 minutes previously. These donors – called non-heart-beating (or asystolic) donors – are people who have died very suddenly, usually from a heart attack. Their hearts have stopped beating, and they are dead. They have not necessarily been put on a life support machine.

Patients who have kidneys from non-heart-beating donors are quite likely to have a period of dialysis after the transplant. This does not normally affect the long-term results.

Patients who are offered a transplant can ask whether it is from a heart-beating or non-heart-beating donor. They have a right to know this, even though they will not be told any other details about the donor. After receiving a cadaveric kidney, patients may write to the donor's family, via the transplant co-ordinator, if they wish, but it is essential that both donor and recipient remain anonymous. Patients should feel free to discuss these issues with their transplant co-ordinator after the transplant.

If someone is on the national waiting list (see *below*) for a cadaveric kidney, they can still ask a relative, partner or friend to give them a kidney. These living related (and unrelated) transplants are described more fully in *Chapter 12*. It is not as important to have a well-matched transplant if the donor is a living person (see *page 86*).

XENOTRANSPLANTATION

The term 'xenotransplantation' refers to the possibility of using organs (such as kidneys) taken from animals (especially pigs) for transplantation into humans. A certain amount of research has been done in this area, but the problems are currently considered to be too great. One major concern is the risk of passing on animal viruses to humans.

STEM CELL 'KIDNEYS'

Research is also being carried out to see if kidneys can be grown or repaired using stem cells. These are very simple cells taken from an adult (or human fetus) that can be programmed to grow into more mature (kidney-like) cells.

Although this research has received considerable publicity, and might change the face of kidney failure in years to come, it is doubtful it will help people with kidney failure in the near future.

THE TRANSPLANT WAITING LIST

At present, not enough cadaveric kidneys are donated to meet the demand. Changes in seat-belt laws and improvements in medicine mean that fewer people now die from the accidents or illnesses that would have made them suitable donors.

So people who are waiting for a cadaveric kidney are put on to a waiting list. Their details, including their blood group and tissue type, are put onto a national computer at United Kingdom Transplant (UKT) in Bristol. When surgeons remove two kidneys from a patient who has died, UKT finds the most suitable patient for each kidney – either locally or in the rest of the country.

A nationally agreed 'scoring system' decides where the kidneys go. It is based on a combination of blood group and tissue type matching, and the length of time the patient has been on the waiting list, and some other factors. Even though it is as fair as it can be, some patients are disadvantaged – especially Asian people. This is partly because Asian people have different blood groups from white people, and there are fewer suitable Asian donors. It is particularly important therefore for Asian patients to find a living donor in their family, as they may have to wait a very long time to get a cadaveric kidney in the UK.

The waiting list works on the basis of finding the 'right' dialysis patient for the 'right' kidney, when one becomes available. It does not work on a 'first-come, first-served' basis. Transplants are allocated to the patient who is the best match for the kidney in terms of blood group and tissue type. In other words, the patient does not join a queue, knowing that his or her name will come up after a reasonably fixed time. It is not really a waiting list, more of a register. The average waiting time for a transplant is about 2 years. It is important to note that this is an average: it can be 2 days, or 20 years – or never.

It may sometimes be necessary to take a patient off the transplant list. This may be done, for example, if someone develops a serious infection or a heart problem, or if they need a major operation. The decision is not made lightly. Any patient whose name is removed from the list should be told about the decision, and informed whether removal from the list is temporary or permanent. Patients who are unsure whether or not they are 'on the list' should ask their kidney doctor or nurse. They can also ask their unit staff to inform them if their name is ever taken off the waiting list.

BEING READY FOR A TRANSPLANT

Patients who are on the waiting list for a transplant will not be given very much notice that a kidney is available for them. So they need to be prepared to go to the hospital at short notice. Some patients are given a 'bleep' so that they can be contacted more easily. It may be sensible to invest in a mobile phone and leave it on 24 hours a day. If you take a holiday outside the UK, you may miss a call when a kidney becomes available.

When patients are on the transplant waiting list, it is largely up to them to make themselves contactable at all times, day and night. If a patient cannot be found, the kidney will be offered to someone else. When a patient 'gets the call', they should go to the hospital at once and not have anything to eat or drink (in preparation for the anaesthetic).

TESTS BEFORE THE OPERATION

Patients called in to the hospital for a transplant are not guaranteed to receive it. Before the operation can go ahead, it is necessary to check that the patient is well enough to have the operation, and that they will not reject the transplant kidney:

1. Physical examination. The patient is first given a thorough physical examination by a doctor. The purpose of this is to check that it is safe to proceed with the operation. For example, if a patient has a heavy cold, it may considered too much of a risk for them to have an anaesthetic. If the patient 'fails' this assessment, they will be sent home, and put back on the waiting list.

2. The cross-match. This test is the final hurdle before the operation. The cross-match is a blood test that checks the patient has no antibodies (substances that normally help the body to fight infection) that would react with the donor kidney. High levels of such antibodies in the blood mean that the new kidney is likely to be rejected as soon as it is put into the patient, even if it seems a good match.

A cross-match is done by mixing a sample of the patient's blood with blood cells from the donor. If there is no reaction (i.e. if the patient's blood does not start attacking the donor's cells), it is assumed that the patient will be less likely to reject the new kidney when it is transplanted. This is called a negative cross-match, and means that the operation can go ahead.

If the cross-match is positive (i.e. there is a reaction between the patient's blood and the donor's cells), the patient will be sent home and put back on the waiting list. This can be very disappointing, but it is much better to return to dialysis for a while than to be given a kidney that doesn't work, and which may make the recipient extremely ill.

THE TRANSPLANT OPERATION

Undergoing an operation to have a kidney transplanted is a major procedure, and afterwards all patients have to take certain medicines and other precautions for the rest of their lives. This applies whether the transplanted kidney was from a cadaveric donor or from a living donor. More details about the operation itself, and life after transplantation, are given in *Chapter 13*.

KEY FACTS

1 For the right patient at the right time, a transplant is the best treatment for kidney failure.

2 If a transplant works well, you will be totally free from dialysis, able to eat and drink normally and continue working. Your sex life may also improve.

3 Suitability for a transplant is more important than age. Up to 40% of patients with kidney failure may be suitable to receive a transplant.

4 Transplants are matched to individual patients in terms of blood group and tissue type.

5 Transplant kidneys come from three sources: cadaveric transplants, living related transplants and living unrelated transplants.

6 The transplant waiting list works on the basis of finding the 'right' kidney for the 'right' person – i.e. patients do not join a queue.

7 Patients have to wait on the transplant waiting list for an average of about 2 years. Asian or Black patients may have to wait longer, so should certainly consider a living transplant if a suitable donor is available.

8 Patients who are called into hospital to receive a kidney transplant need to undergo a series of tests before the operation to make sure the kidney is suitable for them.

12 LIVING DONOR TRANSPLANTATION

In this chapter we discuss the issues surrounding living donor transplantation, the procedures and processes involved, the benefits of this type of transplant, and some of the possible problems.

INTRODUCTION

The first successful kidney transplant was a living donor transplant. It was performed on 23 December 1954 by Joseph Murray and his team at the Peter Bent Brigham Hospital, Boston, USA. A kidney was removed from one man and transplanted into his genetically identical twin brother.

In the UK, the majority of kidneys for transplantation are donated by people who have died (cadaveric transplants). However, a significant proportion (in 2004, this was 28% in the UK) are donated from a relative or someone close to the person who has kidney failure. Human beings do not need two kidneys – quite why we have a 'spare one' is not known. The loss of one kidney will not usually cause any harm to the donor, providing the other one is healthy and functioning. The proportion of living transplants is increasing every year. In some UK units, it now accounts for as many as 40% of all transplant operations. These rates match the European 'leader' in living transplantation, Sweden, where 38% of all kidneys transplanted in 2004 came from living donors. In countries, such as Japan, where cadaveric transplantation is almost unheard of for cultural reasons, living transplant offers the only real option to coming off or avoiding dialysis.

A transplant from a living donor can have many benefits. For most patients, the possibility of a transplant kidney from a living donor will be the best chance of having a transplant operation before dialysis is needed. If a loved one is donating a kidney, the whole transplant procedure will be planned, and both donor and recipient are usually well prepared for the operation.

However, there are risks with the procedure. Just as with a cadaveric transplant, the kidney may not work – in fact, 1 in 20 living transplants are not working a year after the transplant operation. So it is worth considering the emotional aspects of living transplantation before embarking on the process. Both you and the donor need to talk about the possibility of complications following the operation, and how you might feel if the transplant doesn't work.

A growing number of units now have a transplant co-ordinator whose main job is to organise living transplants. This is part of the reason why these transplants are becoming more common.

Anyone who is on the list for a cadaveric transplant can have a live transplant if they have a suitable donor.

THE BENEFITS (AND HOW LONG THEY LAST)

Accepting a kidney from a loved one means that the wait for a transplant may be shorter than the wait for a cadaveric transplant. In some circumstances, the transplant may take place before you need to start dialysis. The transplant operation can also be planned, on a date which is suitable for everyone involved, whereas cadaveric transplants often happen at very short notice.

A kidney from a live donor is likely to function for longer than a cadaveric kidney. In 2004, in the UK, 94% of living donor transplants were still working after the first year (that is more than 19 out of 20), 85% after 5 years and 60% at 10 years. This is in contrast to only 88% of cadaveric transplants at one year (about 18 out of 20), 73% at 5 years, and 46% after 10 years after a transplant.

These statistics are all very well, but anyone considering accepting a kidney from a living donor will want to know how long a living transplant will last for *them*. As with a cadaveric kidney (see *page 80*), any individual living donor transplant may last 5 minutes or 20 years, or indeed it may not work at all. But, on average, a living donor transplant will last 12 years (that is 5 years of 'extra kidney life' when compared to a cadaveric kidney).

No one really knows why a living donor transplant usually lasts longer than a cadaveric one – particularly since the tissue type is usually less well matched to that of the person receiving the transplant. Certainly, a kidney being transplanted from a living donor is usually of better quality than a cadaveric kidney.

This is because living donors are carefully screened for any diseases that might affect their kidneys, such as hypertension or diabetes. The donor's kidneys are also checked to make sure that they function perfectly, and are not likely to fail in the future. Also, a living transplant is more likely to be done before dialysis because it is often one of the first avenues the consultant will 'explore' when a patient is first diagnosed. So the patient does not have to experience the stress of dialysis on blood pressure and the heart.

Also, the time in which the kidney is outside a human body after it has been removed from the donor (i.e. 'still fresh') – called the cold ischaemia time – seems to be a crucial factor. This is less than 1 hour for a live transplant, but 12–36 hours (the average is 20 hours) for a cadaveric transplant. The benefits of transplanting the kidney as soon as possible after it is removed from the donor seem to be much more important than other issues such as tissue type for the success of the transplant.

A living donor transplant may improve the relationship between donor and recipient, as there is a common bond between the two. However, relationships can be complicated and this may not always be the case. There is also some evidence to suggest that the recipient of a living donor transplant is more likely to take the medication required after the transplant, perhaps because the recipient feels more of a responsibility towards the new kidney.

If your kidney failure is diagnosed at an early stage, you could be considered for live kidney transplant up to 6 months before you need dialysis. At this point your creatinine level is likely to be about 400 µmol/l (micromoles per litre of blood). If you already have a transplant that is starting to fail, you could have a live transplant before you need to return to dialysis. But this is up to your own kidney unit's individual policy.

PATIENT SURVIVAL AFTER LIVING DONOR TRANSPLANTS

There is some evidence from the USA that patients who have a living donor transplant will live longer than those receiving cadaveric transplants – having a 98%, 92% and 81% chance of being alive at 1, 5 and 10 years after the transplant, if the transplant is still working. Although there are some problems with this data, remember that there is a 95%, 86% and 67% chance for a patient with a cadaveric transplant at the same time points.

SURVIVAL AFTER TRANSPLANTS: COMPARISON TO DIALYSIS

These survival rates may not seem that good (either for living donor or cadavaric transplants), as most patients have their transplant when they are quite young. But these numbers should be compared with what would happen if the patient stayed on dialysis. For example, 20–25% of patients are dead within 1 year of starting dialysis. This is a not an entirely fair comparison, as transplant patients are younger and so would be expected to live longer. While doctors may not necessarily believe transplants are more likely than dialysis to improve survival for patients with kidney failure, there is general agreement that they can offer a better quality of life.

CADAVERIC OR LIVING DONOR TRANSPLANT – WHICH IS BEST?

It is difficult to give firm advice about which is the 'best' type of transplant, even though there are clear medical benefits of a living donor transplant to the recipient. These benefits, outlined above, are in terms of the likelihood of both the kidney working and the patient being alive at 5 and 10 years after a transplant. There are, however, significant risks to the donor. Nonetheless, it is the view of the authors that if both sides are willing, and understand and accept the risks, then it is 'better' for most patients that their first transplant is a living donor transplant. This is especially important in families, such as Asian and Black families, where a suitable cadaveric kidney is likely to be harder to come by. If this first transplant ever fails, they should then have another living donor transplant, or a cadaveric transplant. Not all people, however, would agree with this view.

In the end, it is up to each donor and recipient pair to make the decision, having taken in the type of information put forward in this chapter, and discussed this with their doctors and the rest of their family.

WHO CAN DONATE A KIDNEY?

Almost anyone can donate a kidney to a loved one. The best donor is an identical twin, as the tissue type is identical. Unfortunately, most people do not have an identical twin waiting to give them a kidney. A kidney from a non-identical twin may also be suitable, but again, few patients have non-identical twins. If a kidney patient has a friend, partner or relative who is at least 16 years old, healthy, and willing to give them a kidney, they should speak to the transplant co-ordinator (or other senior nurse or doctor) at their unit.

The most suitable donor is usually a brother, sister, father, mother, son or daughter, but other more distant relatives may be suitable – uncle, aunt, nephew, niece, cousin, grandparent or grandchild. In fact, the donor does not necessarily have to be a blood relative. The patient's wife, husband, partner or close friend may also be suitable. About 50% of people, blood relatives or otherwise (if they are fit), may be suitable to donate a kidney to any given patient.

As human beings do not need two kidneys to be healthy, the donor is unlikely to come to any harm by losing a kidney. However, even if a kidney comes from a loved one, it is important that both the donor and the patient understand that the kidney is not guaranteed to work.

However, there are some situations where it would not be possible for a living person to donate a kidney. These include potential donors with the following conditions:

- HIV or AIDS-related infection;
- hepatitis B or C infection;
- major heart or breathing problems;
- diabetes (either type);
- significant kidney disease;
- most cancers;
- very high blood pressure;
- intravenous drug abuse;

- extreme obesity;
- pregnancy;
- having only one kidney;
- evidence of financial or non-financial coercion;
- inability of a potential donor to give informed consent; or
- age below 16 years.

In addition, doctors would think very seriously before allowing anyone to donate a kidney if any of the following applied:

- age over 70 years;
- age below 18 years;
- intellectual impairment but able to give informed consent;
- mild obesity;
- family history of diabetes;
- psychiatric disorders; or
- mild high blood pressure.

WHICH DONOR?

Sometimes, when patients are told they will need a transplant to treat their kidney failure, they can be inundated with offers from their family and friends. Each potential living donor will be assessed for their medical suitability to donate a kidney, and to ensure they are well both before, during and after the operation. If more than one person is a suitable donor, it can be difficult to decide which one to accept a kidney from.

But if a patient has a parent and a brother or sister, both of whom are willing (and able) to donate, it might be 'better' to accept the kidney from the parent now, and then 'keep' the sibling's kidney for later in life, if the first transplant ever fails. However, there are no hard and fast rules. The situation will vary between different patients; each individual will have different relationships with the various members of their family circle, and will not necessarily feel closest to their nearest blood relative.

There is no evidence that a woman of child-bearing age (provided she is not actually pregnant at the time) will be at any more risk than anyone else who is offering to be a donor. Nor is there any evidence that it will affect her chance of getting pregnant, or put a future pregnancy at risk.

WHO WILL DO THE ASKING?

It is up to kidney patients to ask their friends or family to see if they are willing to donate a kidney. Doctors will not usually ask a patient's loved ones for them, but they will talk to anybody who is willing to donate a kidney.

TESTS FOR THE RECIPIENT

These are the same as those outlined in *Chapter 11* (*pages 82–3*).

TESTS FOR THE DONOR

As with a cadaveric transplant, the first and perhaps the most important test, to see if the potential transplant might work, is a simple blood test to find out the blood group of the donor. Usually, if the patient's blood group and the donor's blood group are not compatible (according to the rules outlined on *page 79*), no further tests will be carried out. The transplant is unlikely to go ahead, so the transplant tests will be stopped.

Some units are now introducing a new technique called desensitisation which is making successful transplants more likely when a donor is in the 'wrong' group.

If the test is all right, blood samples will be taken to test the donor's liver and kidney function. If these prove satisfactory, the next stage of the screening process can then go ahead.

The donor will need to have a thorough medical examination. This is usually done by two separate doctors – a kidney doctor (usually a different one from the doctor responsible for the patient), and the surgeon who will perform the operation. The doctors will check to make sure that the donor has a normal blood pressure. If their blood pressure is found to be high, the doctors will monitor it for 24 hours – this is because it may only be high at certain times of the day or in certain circumstances. In some cases, the doctors may still agree to go ahead with the transplant, even if the donor has high blood pressure, just as long as it is well controlled using only one type of blood pressure tablet.

An ultrasound scan will then be used to make sure that the donor has two kidneys, and that both are functioning equally well. The function of the individual kidneys can be assessed by a test such as nuclear medicine test (see page 48). Each kidney should be providing 50% of the total kidney function. It is no good if one kidney is undertaking 70% of the work while the other kidney only does 30% of the work. If the surgeon then removed the kidney that did 70% of the work, this could be disastrous for the donor.

The potential donor will also have an ECG (a heart trace, see page 151) and a chest X-ray to ensure there are no problems with their heart or breathing. They may also be given an exercise tolerance test to see how their heart reacts under light exercise.

Blood tests will be carried out for infections such as HIV and hepatitis B and C. Blood samples will also be used to test the donor's genetic compatibility with the recipient (tissue type). This is necessary for all live related transplants so that the genetic relationship between donor and recipient can be proven. Tissue matching is also undertaken in live unrelated transplantation to find out if the donor and recipient are well matched. However, as discussed above (page 80), close matching is not necessary in living transplants.

In addition, there will also be a cross-match test (as in cadaveric transplantation) between donor and recipient. As with cadaveric transplantation, if the cross-match is negative, this means the transplant work-up can continue, but if the cross-match is positive, the transplant cannot go ahead.

Most units also carry out a psychological assessment of both donor and recipient. This is to make sure that both are happy about the procedure, and the effects it may have on them and their families. The psychologist will make sure that both people are able to cope if the transplant fails or anything happens to either the donor or the recipient.

Finally, to help the surgeons decide which kidney (left or right) to remove, the blood vessels to each kidney must be examined using either a type of computed tomography (CT) scan that takes a special look at the blood vessels to the kidneys (a CT angiogram), or a normal renal angiogram. The CT angiogram is safer but does not produce quite such good pictures.

LIVING UNRELATED TRANSPLANTS

Most living donor transplants are performed using kidneys from people who are related to each other, such as genetically related family members. These are called living related transplants (LRTs).

However, an increasing number of live kidney transplants use the organs from people who are not genetically related to each other, although they do have a 'relationship' with each other. This could either be through marriage, co-habitation or a long-standing friendship. Whatever the circumstances, before any live transplant can go ahead, the relationship must be proven. These are called living unrelated transplants (LURTs).

If the donor and the recipient are from the same family, the relationship can be proved from blood samples. If the relationship is an emotional one (husband, wife, partner or friend), it must be proved in other ways. In these situations, each case must be reported to the Unrelated Living Transplant Regulatory Authority (ULTRA), an authority regulated by the Department of Health. ULTRA's role is to ensure that the kidney is being donated freely and for no other reason than to benefit the recipient's health. ULTRA has a panel of members consisting of a medical director and two elected lay members, all of whom will assess the suitability of each individual application.

ULTRA can only authorise the transplant if the relationship can be proven. The doctors looking after the potential recipient and donor have to prepare a report for ULTRA to support the proposed reason for the transplant. An independent third party specialist doctor, who is not involved with the care of either the recipient or the donor, will also need to submit a report. This doctor must interview both people separately and together in order to prepare the report. The reports need to be supported by documentary evidence such as a marriage certificate, photographs of the donor and recipient together, or evidence of co-habitation.

Although it only usually takes about 2 weeks for ULTRA to grant permission for the transplant to go ahead, collecting all the evidence may take much longer.

BUYING AND SELLING ORGANS

In the UK, it is illegal to buy or sell kidneys for transplant. There must be no pressure put on to any potential donor to donate, or recipient to accept. It is also illegal for a person (no matter how well meaning) to donate a kidney to a stranger.

Even though it is illegal to offer payment to enable the live transplant to take place, it *is* legal for the donor to be repaid reasonable costs incurred due to travelling (even from abroad) or loss of earnings. This facility is included in the Human Organ Transplant Act (1989). The renal social worker should know how to obtain this money from the Health Authority or Primary Care Trust.

BEING OFFERED A CADAVERIC TRANSPLANT WHILE PLANNING A LIVING DONOR TRANSPLANT

If the patient is on the cadaveric waiting list, and is having the necessary tests for a living transplant, they may be lucky enough to be offered a cadaveric organ. They will then have to make the difficult decision whether or not to accept the organ. This decision is made harder by the fact that it is possible that the living transplant may have better results. If the cadaveric organ is not a good match, or it is not a particularly 'good' organ, it may be better to say 'no', and proceed with the living transplant. But ultimately, the decision is a personal one for the patient to discuss with their family, the donor and the doctors.

PREPARATION FOR A LIVING DONOR TRANSPLANT

The length of time it takes to prepare the donor and recipient for a live kidney transplant can vary from one unit to another, depending upon a variety of factors:

- The process will be quicker if there is a full-time dedicated live transplant co-ordinator.

- The process may be delayed if it is necessary for either donor or recipient to have additional pre-transplant tests as a result of initial screening.

- If the donor is not a blood relative of the recipient, it will be necessary to contact ULTRA for permission to carry out the operation. This usually takes about 2 weeks, athough getting all the necessary information together can take considerably longer.

On average, it can take around 3–6 months to prepare for a living donor transplant. Sometimes, the time is deliberately long so as to give both parties sufficient time for careful consideration.

It is important that the donor allows for time off work before the transplant as well as after, so that the relevant tests can all be done.

REMOVING THE KIDNEY FROM THE DONOR

There are two ways a live kidney can be donated, either by open surgery, or laparoscopically (using keyhole surgery). The removal of a kidney is called a nephrectomy:

1. Open nephrectomy. Open surgery is the more usual method of removing the kidney. The surgeon makes a cut from the middle point of the side of the chest to the side of the abdomen. Part of a rib may also need to be removed. This method leaves a much larger scar than keyhole surgery. It also takes longer for the donor to recover after the operation. However, using conventional surgery significantly reduces the risk of complications during the operation.

2. Laparoscopic nephrectomy. Some kidney units remove the kidney using keyhole surgery. A small cut is made above the pubic hairline (a 'bikini' or 'low bikini' cut). The kidney is located and removed with the help of a small camera that helps the surgeon to see inside the body without cutting the patient right open. The benefit of this procedure is that the patient has a smaller scar and a quicker recovery time. But there are some disadvantages. There is an increased risk of complications, such as potential damage to the kidney being donated.

Whichever method is used to remove the kidney, the surgeon takes great care not to damage the organ in any way. The surgeon also removes the blood vessels and tubes surrounding the kidney, as they will be used for the recipient.

If the kidney is removed using laparoscopic nephrectomy, the donor will be in hospital for about 3–5 days, but after open surgery this could be 6–9 days.

How soon the donor returns to work will depend on the type of work and their general fitness before the operation. If the work is physically demanding, the donor will probably need a longer recovery time than someone who has sedentary work.

If the kidney is donated by laparoscopic nephrectomy, the donor can probably return to work within 3–4 weeks of the operation. With open surgery, it is advisable to remain off work for about 12 weeks.

RISKS TO THE DONOR

Although any surgical procedure carries with it a small risk (there is about a 1 in 2,000 risk of dying as a result of any operation), the risks to a healthy donor should be minimal if all the pre-operative tests have been carried out. The donor should be aware, however, that the more invasive tests (such as the angiogram) do themselves carry some risk. Anyone who donates a kidney will be seen regularly after the operation. Most units recommend kidney donors should be seen by a kidney specialist every year for life. There is some evidence to suggest that kidney donors live longer than other people on average – nobody knows why this might be so.

There will be some pain and discomfort after the operation, which should get better after a few days. One in 25 patients, however, get long-term pain in the site of the wound. This can usually be controlled by injections given from time to time.

There is usually a 10–20% rise in the donor's creatinine level after losing a kidney.

Some donors may experience protein in their urine (proteinuria) after the operation, and about 10% of all donors may develop high blood pressure. This is the same as the incidence of high blood pressure within the general population.

A major problem of donating a kidney to a loved one is the potential emotional upset if a live transplant fails at an early stage.

RISKS TO THE RECIPIENT

For the recipient, a live kidney transplant operation carries the same risks it would do for a cadaveric transplant (see *page 96*).

Also (as mentioned on *page 78*) some patients may find their original disease, especially a type of glomerulonephritis called focal and segmental glomerulonephritis (FSGS), may return in a transplanted kidney. This is a problem in both cadaveric and live transplants, but will not necessarily cause the transplant to fail.

REJECTION

Unless the live transplant has come from a genetically identical donor (an identical twin), there will be a risk of rejecting the kidney. Around 40% of patients may experience rejection at some point in the first year after a transplant (not necessarily leading to loss of the kidney). This is about the same as the risk for people who have had a cadaveric transplant. It means that it is very important for patients to take their immuno-suppressant medication very carefully, to help avoid this problem. More information about rejection and immuno-suppressant medication is given in the following chapter.

CONCLUSION

Living donor transplants are becoming more common in the UK, but there is still a large shortfall in the number of kidneys available. Hopefully, with better awareness of the higher success rate of live transplants, the number will continue to rise.

KEY FACTS

1 Although the majority of kidneys transplanted in the UK are from people who have died, around 28% are given by a living relative, partner or friend of the patient.

2 All would-be donors will be carefully assessed to ensure they are fit enough to donate a kidney. Nonetheless, there are risks to both the donor and recipient.

3 Most live donors are related to the patient (LRTs), but an increasing number of kidneys are now being given by partners or friends (LURTs).

4 Live unrelated transplants (LURTs) cannot take place without authorisation from ULTRA, the Unrelated Living Transplant Regulatory Authority.

5 Benefits of live transplants include shorter waiting times and the potential for advance planning. The kidneys are likely to last longer than cadaveric ones, and the patient also has a better chance of living longer after a live transplant than after a cadaveric transplant.

6 It is illegal to buy or sell kidneys for a transplant in the UK.

7 If you have a living donor transplant, the risk that your body will reject the new kidney is still there, as for any other transplant patient. So you, too, will have to take immuno-suppressant drugs very carefully, for the rest of your life.

13 THE TRANSPLANT OPERATION AND AFTER

This chapter describes what happens during a kidney transplant operation, and what to expect afterwards. The importance of continuing treatment, and possible side effects of drugs, are addressed.

INTRODUCTION

Transplanting a kidney is a straightforward operation, with a good success rate. The principles have not changed much since the 1950s, when the first kidney transplants were being pioneered in America. After a transplant, patients will need to take drugs daily for the rest of their lives. If a transplant fails, patients can go back to dialysis or possibly have another transplant.

THE TRANSPLANT OPERATION

An operation to transplant a kidney requires a general anaesthetic and lasts about 2–3 hours. The surgeon makes a diagonal incision (cut) into the abdomen, on the right or the left, below the navel (see *page 95, diagram 1*).

The patient's own kidneys are usually left in place. The transplant kidney is placed lower down in the abdomen, just above the groin (see *page 95, diagram 2*). The transplant kidney has its own artery (to take blood to it), vein (to take blood from it) and ureter (to take urine to the bladder).

The artery belonging to the new kidney is attached to the patient's main artery supplying blood to the leg on that side of the body. The vein belonging to the new kidney is attached to the main vein carrying blood from that leg. These leg blood vessels are big enough to be able to send blood to and from the new kidney without affecting the blood supply to the leg. The transplant kidney's ureter is attached to the patient's own bladder. A small plastic pipe (called a double J stent) is usually inserted into the ureter (see *page 95, diagram 3*) to help prevent the ureter from becoming blocked after the operation. At the end of the operation, the patient's abdomen is closed with stitches.

POST-OPERATIVE TUBES

Patients waking up from the anaesthetic after the transplant operation, will find they will have several tubes coming out of them. These will include:

- a urinary catheter (a tube into the bladder);

- a central venous pressure (CVP) line (which is placed under the collar bone or in the side of the neck, and measures the pressure of blood inside the heart);

- an intravenous drip in the arm (to give the patient fluid and drugs if necessary); and, probably,

- one or more surgical drains coming out of the abdomen (to drain off any fluid that gathers around the kidney after the operation).

These tubes will be removed one by one over the next few days. The urinary catheter is usually left in place for 5 days or more. The double J stent is usually removed during a small operation (under local or general anaesthetic) about 3 months after the transplant. PD patients may also have their catheter removed at the same time. Some haemodialysis patients find their fistula stops working at some stage after the transplant. This does not matter, provided the transplant is working well.

AFTER THE OPERATION

The first few days after the operation are critical, and patients are monitored very closely. Particular attention is paid to blood pressure, fluid intake and urine output. Most patients are able to drink and eat small amounts and also to sit out of bed the day after the operation.

Patients will have their blood creatinine level measured every day. This shows whether or not the transplant kidney is working. The amount of urine that the new kidney makes is not a reliable indicator, as people who have just had a transplant may produce a large volume of urine that does not contain many toxins. In about one third of kidney transplant patients (more if the kidney has come from a non-heart-beating donor – see *page 81*), the kidney does not produce any urine in the first few days (and sometimes weeks) after the transplant. This does not mean that the transplant will never work. If the transplant does not work at the start, patients will need to continue dialysis and play a waiting game until the kidney starts working.

- **A 'good transplant' is one that is working well after 1 year, not 2 weeks.**

Patients will usually stay in hospital for about 2 weeks. After leaving hospital, they will need to go to the clinic very frequently for many months, initially 2–3 times per week, then once a week, then once every 2 weeks, and so on. When the doctors are satisfied that the kidney is working well, the patient's appointments may be extended to once every 3 months or so.

It usually takes 3–6 months for patients who have had a kidney transplant to return to normal activities, including work. Transplant patients are recommended not to drive for at least 1 month after the operation. The function of the kidney, and the risk of infection, will not be affected by having sex. However, it is probably best not to resume sexual activity until about 4 weeks after leaving hospital.

HOW LONG WILL THE TRANSPLANT LAST?

A kidney transplant does not last for ever. The average lifespan of a transplanted kidney is around 7 years for a cadaveric kidney, and about 12 years for a living related transplant. The average for a living unrelated transplant is somewhere between the two. So the 'best' (longest-lasting) kidney transplant is one from a relative, then a friend or partner, then a dead person. There is more information about the length of time you can expect a kidney transplant to last in Chapters 11 and 12.

Another way of looking at how long a transplanted kidney is likely to last is to look at the percentage chance that the kidney will be working at set time points. A transplanted cadaveric kidney has, on average:

- a 90% chance of working 1 year after the operation;

- a 60% chance of lasting 5 years; and

- a 35% chance of lasting 10 years or more.

The chances that a kidney from a non-heart-beating donor will still be working at the same time points are

Transplant operation

1 Incision sites (see Note below)
2 New kidney position (right side insertion)
3 Double J stent tube (shown in position)

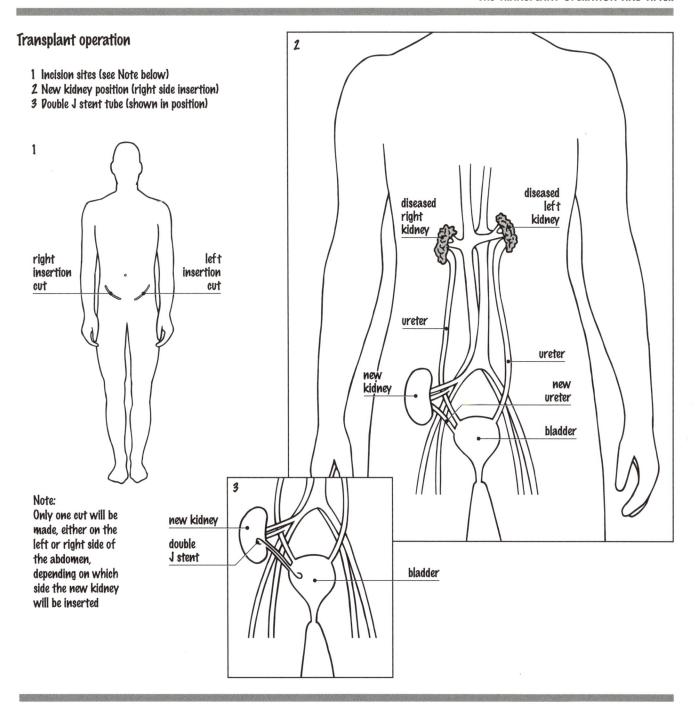

1

right
insertion
cut

left
insertion
cut

Note:
Only one cut will be
made, either on the
left or right side of
the abdomen,
depending on which
side the new kidney
will be inserted

2

diseased
right
kidney

diseased
left
kidney

ureter

ureter

new
kidney

new
ureter

bladder

3

new kidney

double
J stent

bladder

similar. The chances that a kidney donated by a living person will be working at these times are higher – on average:

- a 95% chance of working 1 year after the operation;
- a 70% chance of lasting 5 years; and
- a 55% chance of lasting 10 years or more.

Younger patients may need two or more transplants in their lives. If a transplant fails, the patient can restart dialysis, and most can go back on the transplant waiting list.

POSSIBLE PROBLEMS AFTER A TRANSPLANT

Although a transplant is an excellent treatment for most people with ERF, it is not problem-free. Some people who have had a transplant experience a problem called rejection (see below). Rejection is part of the reason why transplants do not last for ever.

Other problems that a patient may experience after a transplant include drug side effects (see page 99), infection (see page 100), heart disease (see page 100) and cancer (see page 100). It must also be repeated that within 1 year of any transplant, around 5% of patients die.

THE REJECTION PROCESS

'Rejection' means that the patient's body recognises that the transplanted kidney is not 'its own' and tries to 'reject' it from the body. Even when patients and transplant kidneys are apparently 'well matched' (in terms of blood group and tissue type, see pages 79–80), some degree of rejection is common. The severity of rejection varies from patient to patient. Rejection may be either acute or chronic (see page 97).

The body system that is responsible for the rejection process is called the immune system. The immune system is the body's natural defence system. It is located all over the body, and has many different parts. It includes organs (such as the spleen and appendix), lymph nodes (including the 'glands' in the neck) and specialist white blood cells (called lymphocytes).

The usual task of the immune system is to fight foreign invaders. These include germs (such as bacteria and viruses) and foreign objects (such as splinters or thorns embedded in the skin). The immune system also fights cancer. An individual's immune system does not usually attack that person's own cells because these all have a 'friendly face' (consisting of special proteins called antigens on the outer surface of the cells). The immune system recognises the friendly face and knows to leave the cells alone. Germs and foreign objects do not have this friendly face. Nor do cancer cells, which have developed in an abnormal way.

Normally, the immune system is a 'good thing', as it protects the body from dangerous infections, foreign bodies and cancer. However, after a transplant it can be a 'bad thing'. If the immune system recognises that the new kidney does not have the usual friendly face of the body's own cells, it will become overactive and send lymphocytes to attack (reject) the kidney. The body is actually trying to protect you from the kidney, which it perceives as a danger. Luckily, there are drugs – called immuno-suppressant drugs (see page 98) – that can help prevent and treat the rejection process.

ACUTE REJECTION

'Acute' means short term, coming on quickly and needing immediate action. Acute rejection can happen in the first few months (particularly the first few weeks) after a transplant. It is very common – about 40% of patients experience acute rejection in the first year after a transplant. If acute rejection hasn't occurred within 1 year of the operation, then it is unlikely to happen, as long as patients take their drugs correctly. However, if a patient doesn't take their immuno-suppressant drugs, acute rejection can occur at any time. This is why taking these medicines as prescribed, on a regular basis, is so important.

Acute rejection may sometimes cause pain and fever, but usually there are no symptoms. Doctors will suspect that a patient has acute rejection if the blood creatinine level is either not coming down after a transplant, or if it has started to fall and then remains stable or increases again. However, acute rejection is not the only reason why there may be problems with blood creatinine level after a transplant, and these other possibilities are usually looked for first.

● **Investigations**. Tests that might be performed include an ultrasound scan (see *page 49*). This will show whether the patient's ureter (the tube that takes urine from the kidney to the bladder) is blocked. Other possibilities are specialist scanning techniques called a nuclear medicine scan and a Doppler scan. Either of these will show if there are any problems with the blood supply to the new kidney.

The only way to be sure whether a transplant kidney is being rejected is to do a test called a biopsy. This test is described in more detail on *page 46*. It is common for patients who have had a kidney transplant to have two or more biopsies in the weeks after the operation.

A kidney biopsy is an invasive procedure, and therefore there are some risks involved with having one. For more information about the risks involved, see *page 48*.

● **Treatment.** If the biopsy shows signs of rejection, then the patient will usually be given a high dose of a steroid drug, either prednisolone or methylprednisolone. The drug is given by tablet or intravenous injection, once a day for 3 days. These short-course, high-dose treatments are called 'pulses'. Very often, this steroid treatment will suppress the rejection process, and the blood creatinine will start to decrease. Occasionally, a patient may need two courses of this (or a similar) drug.

If pulse prednisolone or methylprednisolone does not work, there are various options. For example, one of the immuno-suppressant tablets may be changed to a similar but slightly 'stronger' drug. An example might be tacrolimus replacing ciclosporin (see *pages 98–9*).

Alternatively, the patient may be given a 5–10 day course of a stronger intravenous injection, such as anti-lymphocyte globulin (ALG), anti-thymocyte globulin (ATG) or orthoclone K T-cell receptor 3 (OKT3) antibody.

These treatments almost always work, and the rejection process goes away. However, all of them can have fairly severe side effects, especially OKT3, which can cause fever, diarrhoea, joint and muscle pain, wheezing, and shortness of breath due to fluid on the lungs (pulmonary oedema).

CHRONIC REJECTION

'Chronic' means long term and of slow onset, not necessarily requiring prompt action. Some doctors think that the term 'chronic rejection' is misleading. The condition it describes is very different from acute rejection. In chronic rejection, there is no real rejection process taking place. The patient's immune system does not attack and reject the transplant kidney in the same way as it does in acute rejection. This is why some doctors call the process 'transplant glomerulopathy' rather than 'rejection'.

Chronic rejection is more like a slow ageing of the new kidney. The cause is uncertain. If it happens, it will usually be more than a year after the transplant operation. Doctors may suspect chronic rejection if a patient's blood creatinine starts to rise slowly after it has been stable for some time. Alternatively, an increasing amount of protein in the urine will be the first sign of chronic rejection. As with acute rejection (see *above*), the only sure way to diagnose the condition is to do a biopsy. There is no treatment for chronic rejection.

The severity of chronic rejection varies. Mild chronic rejection is not usually a problem. However, more severe chronic rejection will eventually lead to failure of the kidney (and therefore a need to go back to dialysis or have another transplant). Chronic rejection may take years to happen, but it is much the most common cause of transplant failure after the first year.

IMMUNO-SUPPRESSANT DRUGS

All patients who have a kidney transplant need to take drugs called immuno-suppressant drugs. As the name 'immuno-suppressant' suggests, the function of these drugs is to suppress the immune system. The aim is to dampen down the immune system sufficiently to stop it rejecting the transplant kidney, while still keeping it active enough to fight infection. Finding the balance can be difficult.

Usually, patients no longer need to continue taking EPO or calcium tablets after a transplant (see *page 33*). However, it is vital for them to take two or three different kinds of immuno-suppressant drugs *every day*. This is because, if they stop taking these drugs, the immune system 'fights back'. If a patient is unable to take these immuno-suppressant drugs, either because they have run out or because they are suffering from diarrhoea or vomiting, they should go to the hospital at once. The immune system does not forget that there is a 'foreign' kidney in the body. It is always waiting for a chance to attack and reject it.

- **If you can't take your immuno-suppressant medicines for 24 hours or more, this is very serious, so go straight to the hospital where you can get appropriate advice.**

Many other medications (both prescribed and 'over-the-counter') can interact with immuno-suppressant drugs, especially with ciclosporin and tacrolimus, both of which are very 'sensitive' drugs. New medications can cause either of these immuno-suppressants to work too well, increasing toxicity, or work less well, risking rejection. Either of these interactions can cause the creatinine level to go up. So patients should always check with the kidney unit pharmacist, or hospital doctor (not their GP, as it is unfair to expect your GP to have this level of specialist knowledge) before taking *any* new medication. Patients should never assume that just because a medicine or tablet is common and easily available (like aspirin, for example), it is necessarily 'safe' to take if they have a transplant.

THE 'BEST' REGIME OF IMMUNO-SUPPRESSANT DRUGS

There is no best regime of immuno-suppressant drugs. Many drugs are now available. However, doctors are now advised (by NICE, see *page 161*) to give patients an injection treatment called basiliximab or daclizumab to suppress their immune system immediately after transplant surgery. This will be given in combination with another drug such as ciclosporin or tacrolimus (FK506). If neither of these prove to be suitable for an individual, alternative drugs, such as sirolimus. One of either azathioprine or mycophenolate mofetil is also usually given. Some people are prescribed steroid drugs such as prednisolone. Other drugs are currently being developed.

If you experience side effects from a particular drug, the drug can be changed for an alternative. Examples might include changing ciclosporin for tacrolimus and vice versa, or azathioprine for mycophenolate mofetil and vice versa.

The choice of drugs is influenced partly by the cost. Also, the long-term side effects of some of the newer drugs are not yet fully understood.

DRUG SIDE EFFECTS

All of the most commonly used immuno-suppressant drugs have their problems:

1. Ciclosporin and tacrolimus. These are the most important drugs used to prevent kidney rejection, and work in a similar way. Unfortunately, if patients are given too much of either, both are toxic (poisonous) to the kidney, this can prevent the transplant from working. This condition is called ciclosporin (or tacrolimus) toxicity. To reduce the risk of problems, patients on either of these will have the amount of the drug in their blood monitored regularly. If problems do occur, these can usually be reversed, either by stopping the drug or reducing the dose. Of course, taking too little of either can increase the risk of rejection. Finding the balance is not easy.

Some patients who take ciclosporin for a long time develop a condition called gum hypertrophy (i.e. swelling of the gums). This is an excessive growth of the gums, which can be unsightly. It is less likely to develop if patients practise good dental hygiene, including regular flossing between the teeth. It the problem becomes severe, the gums can be 'cut back' using a specialist hospital-based dental treatment. Another possible side effect of ciclosporin is excessive growth of hair on the face and body. Tacrolimus does not cause gum swelling or increased hair growth, but can cause hair loss and trembling. Both drugs can cause diabetes, but tacrolimus does so much more often (in up to 30% of patients). If diabetes occurs, it may lead to a lifelong need for insulin injections twice a day.

Both ciclosporin and tacrolimus can also damage the liver and nervous system.

2. Sirolimus. This drug works in a similar way to the above two, but is not so poisonous to the kidney. However, other side effects are seen – especially a very high cholesterol (a type of lipid or fat) level in the blood.

3. Azathioprine and mycophenolate mofetil. The main problem with azathioprine and mycophenolate mofetil is that they can suppress activity in the bone marrow, where blood cells are made. By affecting blood cell production, they can cause a number of serious problems. If too few red blood cells are produced, the patient will suffer from anaemia, causing tiredness. If there are too few white blood cells, the patient will develop a condition called neutropenia. This lack of white blood cells will affect the patient's ability to fight infection. If too few of the blood cells called platelets are produced, the resulting problem is thrombocytopenia, which can cause an increased tendency to bleed.

If you are taking either of these drugs, you may suffer from any or all of the above problems. However, stopping the drug or reducing the dose will normally put matters right. (**NB: this should only be done on advice from your doctor.**)

There are also other side effects. Azathioprine can cause damage to the liver, which will usually be picked up by blood tests. Mycophenolate can cause abdominal pain and diarrhoea.

4. Prednisolone. This drug is a steroid, and, like other steroid drugs, it can cause thinning of the skin (leading to easy bruising) and facial swelling (giving a red and rounded appearance to the face). These problems may lessen if the dose of the drug is reduced.

Like ciclosporin and tacrolimus, prednisolone can also cause diabetes mellitus ('sugar diabetes'). At worst, this might mean that that you would have to take tablets or give yourself insulin injections twice a day. Diabetes can also damage kidneys if it is not well controlled.

A further possible problem with prednisolone is that it can cause crumbling of the joints, especially the hip joints. Pain in either hip, even in the first 3–6 months after a transplant, should be taken seriously. Replacement of one or both hips may become necessary. In the longer term, patients on prednisolone are also at increased risk of thinning of the bones (osteoporosis). Because of this, the vertebrae (bones of the spine) can collapse causing a 'crush fracture'. This can be very painful, as well as reducing your height.

Some doctors try to withdraw steroid tablets after the first 6–12 months because of these side effects on the joints and bones. This usually causes the creatinine to rise by 10 μmol/l (micromoles per litre of blood) or so, which is not usually a problem. But it does carry a very small risk of rejection (or even loss) of the kidney.

INFECTION

Although immuno-suppressant drugs help prevent transplant rejection by making the immune system less efficient, their effect on a patient's ability to fight infections is generally less than might be expected. So people taking immuno-suppressant drugs do not necessarily get one infection after another.

Having said that, there is one infection that is a particular problem after transplantation. It is called cytomegalovirus (CMV) infection. For most people who are not taking immuno-suppressant drugs, CMV is a mild infection that causes a 'flu-like illness. However, in patients who have just received a transplant, CMV infection can be quite a severe illness.

If a transplant patient does ever get CMV, there is a very effective treatment for it. This is called ganciclovir, and is given as a course of injections.

A new virus, the BK virus, has recently been discovered. This can cause the transplanted kidney to function less well, and can also affect the blood. A drug called sidofovir is being used to treat BK virus, although it is not yet known how effective it is. It is given as a course of injections.

HEART DISEASE

Heart attacks and problems with the circulation (such as stroke and reduced blood flow to the legs) are much more common after a transplant. This is partly because of the effects of kidney failure on the circulation before a transplant. It is also due to other new problems after a transplant. These may include high blood pressure, a high cholesterol level in the blood, diabetes (which can start after a transplant, as it is a side effect of many immuno-suppressant drugs) and increased risk of clotting ('thickening') of the blood. The risk of these problems may be reduced if the patient does not smoke, keeps fit, and keeps their weight under control.

If you have had a kidney transplant, you should work with your doctor to keep your blood pressure down (under 120/70 mmHg), your diabetes (if you have it) under control, your cholesterol low (under 5 mmol/l), and perhaps have your blood thinned. This may mean taking more medicines. You may need to take tablets or have insulin injections to control your diabetes. A group of tablets called statins are particularly good at controlling the cholesterol level in the blood. Aspirin can be used to thin the blood, although it will not necessarily be suitable for everyone who has had a kidney transplant.

It is important to ask the doctor why such tablets are not being prescribed, if they are indicated, as having a heart attack or stroke, say 5 years after a transplant, makes it hardly worth the patient going through such a major operation.

CANCER

One of the functions of the immune system is to fight cancer. By making the immune system less efficient to help prevent transplant rejection, immuno-suppressant drugs unfortunately increase the likelihood of getting some types of cancer. A research study has shown that 25% of transplant patients who live for 25 years after a transplant develop some type of cancer.

For example, transplant patients are three times more likely than other people to get skin cancers after a transplant. This makes it very important for people who have had a transplant to use a strong 'sun block' cream to avoid sunburn. Exposure to the sun greatly increases the risk of developing skin cancer. (In Australia, where skin cancer is particularly common, the increased risk to transplant patients rises to 40 times the average.) Provided that skin cancers are diagnosed in good time, they are not usually a major problem. This type of cancer does not usually spread to other parts of the body, and can be easily removed.

Transplant patients are no more likely than anyone else to get the other more common serious problems, such as breast or lung cancer.

LYMPHOMA

A small but significant number (2–5%) of transplant patients develop lymphoma, which is a more serious (leukaemia-like) cancer of the bone marrow and immune system – often within a year of the operation. It is more common in patients who have had stronger immuno-suppressant drugs. About 60% of cases occur in the first year after transplant. The average time from transplant to developing lymphoma is about 9 months. These 'early' cases are particularly serious.

Lymphoma sometimes 'goes away' when the doses of immuno-suppressant drugs are reduced. In more severe cased it has to be treated with high doses of chemo-therapy. In some cases, the immuno-suppressant drugs given for the transplant are stopped, which can lead to loss of the kidney. Although these treatments can be successful, 30–50% of people who develop lymphoma after a transplant die within 2 years of the diagnosis.

KEY FACTS

1 A transplant operation lasts 2-3 hours, and involves staying in hospital for about 2 weeks after the operation.

2 About a third of transplanted kidneys do not work initially, sometimes requiring a short period of dialysis.

3 Up to 40% of patients have at least one episode of acute rejection (of the kidney) after a transplant. These are usually fairly easy to treat.

4 Patients have to take immuno-suppressant drugs daily to prevent their body rejecting a transplant. Not taking them correctly can lead to loss of the kidney. However, these drugs do have side effects.

5 A transplant does not always last for ever. Transplants from living relatives last longest.

6 If a transplant fails, you can go back onto dialysis. Most people can go on to have another transplant.

7 It is important to keep as fit as possible after a transplant. For example, don't smoke, try to keep your weight down, monitor your blood pressure, cholesterol levels and (if you have diabetes) your blood sugar.

8 If you have had a transplant, you will be at greater risk than other people of developing skin cancer, so be extra careful about protecting your skin from the sun. You will also have an increased risk of developing lymphoma, which can sometimes be fatal.

14 DIET

This chapter explains why it is important for people with kidney failure to watch what they eat. It also describes the different dietary advice that they are likely to be given as their condition and treatment change.

INTRODUCTION

One of the questions most frequently asked by kidney patients is, 'Why does the advice given to me about my diet keep changing?' Well, it isn't because the dietitian got it wrong in the first place. The reason is that patients' dietary needs change as their condition changes. So, just as drug therapy and other treatments may need to be altered, diet may also need to be revised to stay in line.

HEALTHY EATING GUIDELINES

It is a good idea for all patients with kidney failure – whether pre-dialysis, on dialysis or with a transplant – to follow 'healthy eating guidelines'.

These guidelines are:

- to eat some high-fibre foods (such as wholemeal bread and cereals);

- to eat only moderate amounts of fats (which should be mainly polyunsaturated); and

- to avoid adding 'extra' salt to foods if you have high blood pressure.

WHAT IS 'NUTRITIONAL STATUS'?

The term 'nutritional status' is used by doctors, nurses and dietitians to describe a patient's state of nourishment. A person with a poor nutritional status is not receiving enough of the right kinds of food. There is no single reliable method of measuring nutritional status: there is no nutritional equivalent of the blood creatinine test (see *Chapter 2*).

Doctors, nurses and dietitians usually assess the nutritional status of their patients with kidney problems by:

- asking how the patient is feeling;

- asking about the patient's diet (perhaps including asking them to keep a record for a while of everything they eat and drink);

- measuring the level of albumin (a type of protein) in the blood (see *page 44*), as a low level of this is linked to malnutrition;

- measuring the size of the patient's muscles; and

- monitoring the patient's body weight.

Research has shown that nutritional status is an important factor in survival. A study of 12,000 haemodialysis patients in the USA showed that patients who had a very low blood albumin when they started dialysis were 17 times more likely to die during the first year of dialysis.

DIETARY PROTEIN AND KIDNEY FAILURE

Protein is an essential nutrient, which enables the body to build muscles, and to repair itself. The main sources of protein in the diet are meat, fish, dairy products and pulses (such as beans and lentils). Everyone – including people with kidney failure – must eat appropriate amounts of protein if they are to avoid serious nutritional problems.

When protein is digested, waste products are formed and enter the blood. One of these wastes is called urea (see page 12). Normal healthy kidneys are quite good at getting rid of urea and other wastes from the blood. However, as kidney failure develops, the kidneys become less and less able to remove wastes from the blood (see Chapter 2). Even so, this does not mean that people with kidney failure should stop eating protein (see below).

DIET BEFORE STARTING DIALYSIS

People with kidney failure who have not yet started dialysis should follow normal healthy eating guidelines. This includes continuing to eat foods that contain protein even after the level of urea in their blood has started to rise.

If people with kidney failure restrict their intake of dietary protein, their urea level will not rise so rapidly. For this reason, it has been suggested that reducing the amount of protein in the diet might delay the need for dialysis. However, such use of protein restriction is controversial, since lower levels of urea in the blood may indicate that patients are becoming malnourished – i.e. they do not receive enough protein to maintain their flesh weight (see page 20).

When the time for dialysis draws closer, some people do not feel as hungry as they used to – and some foods, particularly meat products, may taste 'funny'. Special dietary supplements may help such patients to maintain adequate protein, energy and vitamin intakes. A dietitian will be able to provide advice about these supplements.

DIET DURING DIALYSIS

Several aspects of diet and nutrition are very important for patients on dialysis. All kidney patients are at an increased risk of developing malnutrition (see below).

It may also be necessary to pay special attention to a dialysis patient's intake of phosphate, calcium, potassium, salt, fluid and vitamins (see pages 105–6). In some cases, there may also be other specific individual dietary recommendations (see page 106).

GAINING WEIGHT (OBESITY) AND KIDNEY FAILURE

Even though weight loss is a problem that causes particular concern in kidney failure (see page 104), weight gain can be almost as serious.

Obesity can actually contribute to the development of kidney failure. This is largely because being overweight makes a person much more likely to develop diabetes mellitus, which is one of the major causes of kidney failure.

Reversing obesity (losing weight by dieting) will not cure kidney failure. Nevertheless, the other health advantages, such as reducing blood pressure and strain on the heart, are well worth achieving. At the very least, patients on the transplant waiting list are more likely to cope physically with a transplant operation if they are a healthy weight and do not have raised blood pressure.

More specifically, obesity can cause practical problems for people on dialysis. Overweight people with fat arms can have particular problems with access for haemodialysis. Their veins can be difficult to reach, or weak, and therefore difficult to make a fistula from (see pages 68–9). And PD is less likely to work for patients who have a fat or distended tummy. Very obese patients will be too unfit to be offered a transplant.

If obesity is a problem, healthy eating guidelines may help. Overweight patients should ask to be referred to a dietitian for advice.

LOSING WEIGHT AND KIDNEY FAILURE

Some kidney patients find they lose a lot of weight and become very thin. This is usually because they are not eating enough (especially foods providing protein and energy). Loss of appetite is often one of the first things people notice when their kidneys stop working properly. Such patients rapidly become malnourished.

Malnutrition is the most important, and most dangerous, nutritional problem that can develop in patients on either type of dialysis. So, to prevent malnutrition, patients on dialysis will be asked to increase their food intake (especially their intake of protein).

Doctors are not entirely sure why kidney patients have an increased risk of malnutrition, and why they need extra protein in their diet. A combination of causes seems most likely.

POOR APPETITE AND MALNUTRITION

The most important cause of malnutrition in kidney patients is probably the simplest one – poor appetite. This is one of the major symptoms of kidney failure, and is often the reason why people go to their family doctor in the first place.

When someone is pre-dialysis (or has a failing transplant), worsening of the appetite is one of the reasons why doctors start (or restart) dialysis. When a patient is on dialysis, a change – hopefully an improvement – in their appetite is often the most reliable guide to the effectiveness of the dialysis. It can tell more than any of the blood tests (including the 'key' test, the blood creatinine, see *Chapter 2*).

Dialysis usually restores a kidney patient's appetite to near normal, although few dialysis patients ever really have a 'good' appetite. Dialysis is just not good enough at getting rid of the toxins that suppress appetite. (Doctors do not even know which these toxins are.)

If there is under-dialysis (i.e. a patient is not receiving enough dialysis), loss of appetite is one of the first symptoms of kidney failure to return. An increase in the dialysis dose will then probably help to improve the patient's appetite. However, only a transplant will fully return a patient to a 'normal' appetite.

A build-up of toxins in the blood may not be the only reason for appetite problems in a kidney patient. Severe anaemia (see *Chapter 5*) may also suppress appetite.

Also, PD patients may have a poor appetite because of the dialysis fluid in their abdomen, which can make them feel bloated.

OTHER CAUSES OF WEIGHT LOSS

In addition to appetite problems, a number of other factors may contribute to the increased risk of weight loss in kidney patients on dialysis.

PD patients lose protein and amino acids (substances from which proteins are built up) into their bags of dialysis fluid. Haemodialysis patients also lose amino acids into their dialysis fluid. So kidney patients on both types of dialysis need extra protein in their diet to make up for these losses.

Poor control of blood acidity level (blood tends to be acidic in kidney failure) is another important factor. This is shown by low bicarbonate levels in the blood (see *page 42*). A research study carried out by Dr Stein showed that dialysis patients with higher bicarbonate levels (less acidic blood) were more likely to be alive and better nourished after the first year of dialysis.

Infections also increase a person's requirements for high-protein and high-energy foods, and infections tend to be more common in dialysis patients.

A further possible cause of malnutrition in kidney patients may be that some patients are not eating enough because of dietary restrictions imposed by their doctor or dietitian. Fortunately, such over-zealous dietary restrictions are now going out of fashion.

Loss of weight tends to be more common in haemodialysis than PD patients. PD patients have an extra source of calories – the sugar contained in PD fluid. Some of this is absorbed by the patient, providing the equivalent of approximately 300–500 calories a day – similar to eating between one and two Mars Bars. Haemodialysis patients don't have this extra energy source and may need additional dietary advice and supplements.

PROTEIN/ENERGY SUPPLEMENTS

Protein and/or energy supplements can be very helpful if a kidney patient is not eating enough. These supplements are really very good and supply varying amounts of protein and energy depending on what is needed. The supplements are available on prescription, and hospital dietitians can ask their patients' GPs to prescribe them.

PHOSPHATE AND CALCIUM

Phosphate and calcium are two minerals that affect the health of the bones. When a person has kidney failure, the calcium level in their body tends to be too low, and their phosphate level too high. This puts them at risk of bone problems, due to a condition called renal bone disease (see Chapter 6).

Treatment for kidney patients therefore aims to raise blood calcium levels and also to lower blood phosphate levels. Both these aims can often be achieved by:

- reducing the phosphate content of your diet;

- adequate dialysis if this has been started; and

- using a phosphate binder (calcium carbonate, e.g. Calcichew) taken as tablets with meals.

A low-phosphate diet is not as straightforward as it sounds. It is very difficult to cut down phosphate intake without also lowering protein intake.

Patients who need to adjust their diet to reduce their blood phosphate level will be given specific advice by their dietitian. This will probably include asking them to be careful about eating dairy produce, offal and shellfish – as these all contain particularly high amounts of phosphate. The dietitian may also give advice about the distribution and timing of phosphate-binding tablets.

In general, patients only need to worry about the amount of phosphate in their diet if their doctor or dietitian specifically tells them they have a problem.

POTASSIUM

Potassium is another very important mineral in the human body. The kidneys normally regulate potassium level without any difficulty, but in kidney failure this control is lost. Potassium levels may then be either too high or too low (see Chapter 7, page 41).

The main problem with potassium is that if it rises to a very high (or falls to a very low) level in the blood, it becomes dangerous to the heart, which can stop beating.

Potassium is one of the substances that is measured when dialysis patients have blood tests. Any patient who regularly has high blood potassium levels will get to know their dietitian very well. The dietitian will try to find out if the person is eating anything that might be causing a high level of potassium in the blood.

Many foods contain potassium, but some have more than others. Kidney patients whose blood potassium levels are high or rising will normally be asked to restrict their intake of high-potassium foods. This will involve avoiding some (rather nice) foods, such as chocolate and crisps, and moderating their intake of other potassium-containing foods, such as bananas, oranges and mushrooms. If this dietary restriction does not work, the dietitian may recommend an increase in dialysis dose, usually an increase in the number of hours per haemodialysis session.

PD patients rarely need to restrict their potassium intake, and in fact may sometimes need to increase it.

This is because PD is a continuous process that generally clears potassium from the blood very effectively. Haemodialysis, on the other hand, is an intermittent process. So, in the intervals between dialysis, the blood potassium may begin to rise. These patients may therefore need dietary advice on potassium intake.

Unless their doctor or dietitian tells them otherwise, kidney patients can assume that they do not have a problem with their blood potassium.

WHAT ABOUT SALT AND FLUID?

Salt and fluid advice are often given together. A salty diet may make patients thirsty, and make life very uncomfortable if a fluid restriction is necessary.

Salt restriction usually involves:

- using little or no salt in cooking and at the table; and

- decreasing the intake of high-salt foods, which are mainly convenience and processed foods.

Haemodialysis patients often have greater restrictions on fluid intake than PD patients, and therefore need to be extra careful about salt.

Fluid advice for individual kidney patients is based on a combination of their urine output (if they still pass urine) and the amount of water removed by dialysis. Generally speaking, the more urine patients pass, the more fluid they can drink. A common generalisation is that dialysis patients can drink 500 ml of fluid every day plus the equivalent of any urine they have passed plus any fluid lost by dialysis on the previous day. For many patients, this works out to be about 1 litre for haemodialysis patients and 1.5 litres for PD patients.

VITAMIN SUPPLEMENTS

There are different opinions about the value of vitamin supplements for people who have kidney failure.

Most doctors and dietitians agree that the so-called fat-soluble vitamins (i.e. vitamins A, D, E and K) are rarely a problem and don't need supplementing. Supplements of fat-soluble vitamins may even cause problems, as excessive amounts accumulate in the body. One fat-soluble vitamin – vitamin A (found in large amounts in cod and halibut liver oil capsules) – is known to be toxic and can cause problems if taken to excess.

It is known that the so-called water-soluble vitamins (i.e. vitamins B and C) are lost in both types of dialysis. It is therefore possible that there may be deficiencies if patients reduce their intake of certain foods, either voluntarily or because of potassium restrictions. A case can therefore be made for supplementing these vitamins. But should everyone take supplements, just to make sure, bearing in mind the large number of tablets most kidney patients are taking anyway? Different units adopt different policies.

INDIVIDUAL DIETARY RECOMMENDATIONS

All people with kidney failure are advised, as far as possible, to follow 'healthy eating guidelines' (in brief, to eat a high-fibre, moderate-fat and low-salt diet). In some cases, however, specific individual priorities will over-ride these guidelines.

The most common example of going against the usual guidelines is if someone is losing a lot of weight and needs to boost their intake of calories with fat. In this situation, malnutrition is a more serious and immediate danger than any possible future increased risk of heart disease from a high-fat diet. Hence the reason for the 'unhealthy' compromise on fat intake.

DIET AFTER A TRANSPLANT

A common question after someone has had a kidney transplant is, 'Do I still need to follow a special diet?' The simple answer is, 'No'. If a kidney is functioning well, then there is no need to be on a special diet. If the transplant starts to fail, the situation may be different.

Transplant patients, being immuno-suppressed and at greater risk than other people of picking up infections, should be given information about food hygiene. In addition, they will be advised to follow normal healthy eating guidelines. This is particularly important because of two problems associated with a transplant. Both these problems – excessive weight gain (usually a side effect of taking steroid drugs, such as prednisolone) and high cholesterol levels – increase the risk of heart disease. Healthy eating habits may help reduce the risk.

TAKING CONTROL OF WHAT YOU EAT

Diet is an area where you really can take some control over your lifestyle and feel you are doing something to improve your own situation. Having kidney failure does not mean you have to stop enjoying your food. What it does mean is that you need to understand what you are eating, and learn which foods you can eat as much of as you like; which foods you should have once in a while (as a treat) and which foods you really should consider cutting out altogether. It is important though that, while you follow your doctor and dietitian's advice, you do not become so obsessed with watching the relative values of everything you eat that meals become a chore for you. The Suggested Further Reading list on page 158 will point you in the direction of a couple of books that may help you find the right balance.

KEY FACTS

1 Advice about what you should eat will vary according to the stage of kidney failure you have reached, and the type of treatment you are receiving.

2 'Healthy eating guidelines' – for high-fibre, moderate-fat and low-salt diet – are generally recommended whether you are waiting for dialysis, are on dialysis or have a transplant.

3 It is difficult to measure someone's nutritional state. The blood albumin level is often used, but is not very reliable. A low level may be a sign of malnutrition in some cases.

4 You should only alter your diet when your kidney doctor or dietitian advises you to.

5 Weight gain (obesity) can lead to practical problems if you need haemodialysis or PD. It may also make you so unfit that a transplant operation becomes too dangerous.

6 Weight loss and malnutrition are the major problems for many patients on dialysis – both PD and haemodialysis. So high protein intakes are recommended.

7 If you are on PD, it is unlikely you will need to reduce your potassium intake. But you may need to restrict it if you are on haemodialysis.

8 Eating a lot of salt or salty foods will make you thirsty. You may need to restrict your salt intake, particularly if fluid is restricted.

9 If you have had a transplant, you are unlikely to have any dietary restrictions. But you should try to follow standard healthy eating guidelines.

15 PSYCHOLOGICAL ASPECTS

This chapter looks at the reasons why people with kidney failure may feel differently from people whose kidneys are healthy. It also suggests ways of identifying and coping with the various psychological problems that you may experience.

INTRODUCTION

A diagnosis of kidney failure has a massive impact. It will affect the whole of your life, not just your physical condition. Once you know you have kidney failure, you will have to make changes to the way you live, and learn new skills and coping strategies. You are also likely to find the illness affects the way you feel about yourself, and your priorities in life. What all this means in practice is that the psychological aspects of kidney failure become very important.

BODY AND MIND

Everyone's psychological and emotional well-being has a major impact on their physical well-being. The way you feel will influence the way you behave. Many people eat or drink to cheer themselves up when they feel low, for example. If they are anxious, they may row with their partner. If they don't feel able to manage, they may decide their whole treatment is not worth bothering with.

The way kidney patients behave has a direct effect on their physical condition. They may become less careful about their diet, forget to take their tablets, or abandon fluid restrictions – all of which put additional strain on an already poorly body.

PSYCHOLOGICAL NEEDS

Psychology is about behaviour: why people behave the way they do, and how they can change the way they behave. It is about how people feel about themselves, their situation, the people who are part of their lives. Everybody has psychological needs – not just people who happen to have kidney failure. However old or ill we might be, we all need to be heard, understood and valued. Illness can make this more difficult. People who are unwell may find it hard to express their fears and anxieties, or feel in control of the situation.

STRESSES ON PEOPLE WITH KIDNEY FAILURE

Any long-term or life-threatening illness, can be extremely stressful. Any change – even a pleasant change like getting married – is stressful. When changes are 'negative', however, stress will be greatly increased.

The treatment of kidney failure means you can't avoid changes in lifestyle. People have to adapt their usual routine. They may have to make changes to their eating and drinking habits. They may not have sufficient energy to continue working or to pursue hobbies or interests.

Some of the stresses that commonly affect people with kidney failure are:

- having to make decisions about things they have never even thought about before;
- taking in strange information, to enable them to understand a complex medical subject;
- learning about themselves and the ways they cope with things;
- needing to ask for support to manage their treatment;
- seeing themselves as a complete person, not just as a disease or condition;
- learning to live differently for the rest of their life; and
- worrying about the future.

Changes to the expected progression of life may also cause stress. For example, it may be difficult for a young person to leave home, either because they have kidney failure, or because they feel they should look after a parent with kidney failure. Sometimes people have to cope with unpleasant reactions from their employers and work colleagues. Later in life, retirement may come early and be totally unwelcome.

Other members of the family also have to make adjustments. Kidney failure has an impact on their lives too. The normal pattern of life is disrupted and relationships have to be redefined.

THE DIAGNOSIS

For some people, the diagnosis of kidney failure comes completely out of the blue. This can be extremely difficult to cope with. Even when kidney failure was already suspected, knowing it is definite can cause difficulties. The way that the diagnosis is given, and the quality of support offered immediately afterwards, can make a big difference to a person's future well-being.

INITIAL REACTIONS

Following a diagnosis of kidney failure (or any other serious long-term illness), people typically go through the following stages:

1. Shock. At first, patients (and sometimes also family members and friends) go into a state of shock, feeling stunned, bewildered or strangely detached – as though they are observing life rather than being part of it. This shock can last a short while or may continue for weeks.

2. Grief. Then people begin to react to the news, often with feelings of loss, grief, helplessness and despair. They may feel overwhelmed by reality, and find it difficult to think clearly or plan effectively.

3. Denial. One very common reaction to serious illness is to deny the existence of the disease or its implications. But the problem does not go away, the symptoms get worse, and there are reminders from other people that the illness exists.

4. Acceptance. Gradually, people come to accept reality a little at a time, and begin to make progress towards adapting successfully to their condition.

LONGER-TERM PROBLEMS

Patients with kidney failure often experience longer-term psychological problems too. Some of these are described below:

1. Lack of co-operation with the medical team. Various terms have been used by doctors for 'not doing as you are told'. Until a few years ago, you may have heard the term 'non-compliance' or even 'non-adherence'. Now you are more likely to hear your health professionals using terms such as 'lack of concordance' in relation to an agreed programme of treatment and self-help measures. The term 'concordance' signifies mutual decision making between patient and health professionals. Reasons why patients may find it difficult to keep to the decisions about treatment and lifestyle that have been mutually agreed in this way include:

- they believe that the treatment is not effective, and there is no obvious benefit from it;

- they do not know what effect the treatment is supposed to have, or why it is important to continue with it; and

- the side effects of the treatment are unpleasant.

Almost a third of all patients will have at least one period when they find it difficult to follow the guidance set out by their doctors and nurses – after all, no one likes being told what to do.

You need to be aware, however, that if you don't follow your agreed treatment regime, you can end up very ill indeed. It is much better to learn how to manage your kidney failure by exploring with your doctor or nurse which areas allow you some flexibility, at the same time as being absolutely certain which are the situations where choosing not to follow your treatment plan can be life-threatening. Do talk to your renal unit team. If you understand why you should (or should not) be doing something, you will feel much more motivated about it. Many problems of this nature can be solved by better communication between doctors or nurses and their patients.

2. Anxiety. As well as the anxieties felt by most people at some time in their lives, kidney patients have additional anxieties relating to their condition and its treatment. Some possible problem areas include:

- relationships (e.g. 'We can't share the same interests any more'; 'We've both changed so much');

- quality of life (e.g. 'I miss walking the dog'; 'I'd planned to go abroad');

- employment (e.g. 'I've taken too much time off work');

- practical management (e.g. 'How can I do my CAPD exchanges when I feel so ill?'); and

- understanding (e.g. 'I can't understand all the medical words').

3. Body image. Not all people with kidney failure have problems with their changed body image, but some do. They may see their fistula or PD catheter as a mutilation of their body. They feel horribly scarred and find it really hard to look at themselves.

The perceptions of patients and medical staff can differ widely here. When doctors and nurses talk about a 'really good fistula', they are talking about the ease of access, the rate of blood flow, and the strength of the blood vessels. What the patient experiences is a forearm with a continuous buzzing sensation, and a disfiguring swelling where it used to be smooth and flat. Some patients cannot see their fistula as a 'good' thing at all.

4. Awareness of early death. People with kidney failure know that without treatment they would die. Having to live with this sort of knowledge puts a very different perspective on life's priorities.

5. Dependency and self-confidence. Kidney patients are very dependent – on hospital doctors and nurses, and on their partners, relatives and friends. People with kidney failure have to deal with the fact that their life depends on a machine, on PD bags, or on someone else's kidney. This necessary dependency can undermine a person's confidence in coping with both kidney and non-kidney issues. They may wonder if they are 'doing it right', for example, or worry about becoming dependent on someone they are used to 'taking care of'.

If issues relating to dependency and self-confidence are not dealt with, they may cause conflict between kidney patients and hospital staff or carers.

6. Sense of loss. A person's kidneys have been a part of them since birth. A healthy person will take their kidneys (and every other organ) for granted, never having to think about them. So the failure of this essential body part is likely to give rise to a kind of grieving.

7. Depression. Most people get depressed at some stage in their lives. Periods of depression may be useful, in that they enable people to withdraw from the world for a while, and resolve certain issues. People with kidney failure are no exception. There are times when they feel low, and to do anything at all requires a huge effort; times when they should allow themselves to feel sorry for themselves; and times to cry.

8. Changes to treatment. One of the many difficult things about kidney failure is that the treatment changes over time. For example, patients may change from PD to haemodialysis, or vice versa, or they may receive a transplant, or resume dialysis after a transplant fails.

9. Ageing and bereavement. It is not only a patient's treatment that changes. Everyone changes to some extent as they get older. Tasks that seem easy when someone is young may become more troublesome as the years go by. Coping with kidney failure may become more difficult.

Everyone (perhaps those in perfect health most of all) finds that, as they get older, more and more of their friends will die. This can be a particular problem for older patients in the kidney unit. In addition, if you attend the same unit for a long time, you may see many staff changes. Just as you are building up a rapport with one dialysis nurse, they move to a new job or retire. This can become a strong and supportive relationship and the better it is the more difficult you may find it to adjust to their not being around.

10. Sexual activity. Sexual problems are very common among people with kidney failure and can put strain on a relationship. Concerns about sexual ability vary from person to person. There may be a loss of sex drive, especially in men. For many young men, the most distressing aspect of kidney failure is their inability to get or maintain a normal erection. Women may worry about whether thay can get pregnant, or have a healthy baby. (See *Chapter 16* for more information about sexual problems and fertility.)

11. Conflicting advice. People with kidney failure receive information from lots of different people. The people who pass on this information have themselves already interpreted it according to their own backgrounds and beliefs. So, what a patient hears may not always be totally true. The advice from one source may conflict directly with advice from another. It is not surprising that kidney patients are sometimes confused by what they are told.

Also, what a doctor or nurse tells one patient may not be the same as what they tell another. Every case is different.

12. Poor concentration. Patients sometimes worry that kidney failure may be affecting their brain. They may find that they sometimes cannot concentrate as well, or think as clearly, as they used to before their kidneys failed. These problems may last from a few minutes to several days at a time. However, for most people with kidney failure, most of the time, the ability to concentrate and think clearly is as good as it *ever* was. When there are problems, efficient dialysis will often help a patient to think straight.

FACTORS AFFECTING THE ABILITY TO COPE

Some people cope more easily than others with the psychological and emotional aspects of kidney failure. Research indicates that an individual's ability to cope with illness is influenced by a range of factors.

1. Illness-related factors. The first group of factors relates to the illness itself:

- Some people are more afraid than others of the possible consequences of kidney failure. Fears of disability, disfigurement, pain or early death may need to be addressed. The more they feel threatened by their illness, the harder they will find it to cope.

- Kidney failure often occurs together with other conditions, such as diabetes, anaemia (see *Chapter 5*) and renal bone disease (see *Chapter 6*). These conditions cause their own symptoms, giving kidney patients *even* more things to worry about.

- Some people have to cope with unpleasant side effects from the tablets they must take (particularly if they have had a transplant, see *Chapter 13*).

- The treatment of kidney failure involves major time commitments, which can interfere with finding or holding down a job. Lack of secure employment can be an additional strain.

- Kidney failure requires patients and their families to make changes in their lifestyle. These changes may put pressure on relationships and increase stress.

- Many people with a chronic illness, such as kidney failure, feel self-conscious about their disease and want to hide it from others. This can cause stress and make it harder to cope.

2. Age. The age at which a person develops kidney failure is likely to influence the way they will cope:

- Children may not understand the long-term implications of the condition.

- Adolescents need to be liked and accepted by their peers. Because of this, some may neglect their medical care to avoid appearing different from their friends.

- Young adults with kidney failure may feel they no longer have the chance to develop their lives in the direction they planned – to get married, to have children, or to enter a particular career. Such feelings may cause anger and resentment.

- Middle-aged patients may have problems adjusting to the disruption of an established lifestyle. They may find themselves unable to finish tasks they have started, such as building up a business.

- Older patients may resent not being able to enjoy their retirement.

3. Personality. Aspects of a person's personality can affect their ability to cope with kidney failure:

- People who cope well with long-term health problems tend to have hardy or resilient personalities which allow them to see good in difficult situations. They are able to balance hope against despair and to find purpose in life whatever happens. They maintain their self-esteem and resist feeling helpless and hopeless.

- Kidney failure often means that patients must take on a dependent and passive role, for a while at least. Some people find this especially difficult since it is so different from the independent role they have developed over the years.

4. Social and cultural factors. A person's ability to cope with illness is also affected by their background:

- People from different social, cultural and religious backgrounds will have different ways of dealing with situations. Problems may arise if doctors and nurses fail to take this into account.

- People's beliefs about health come from a number of sources, including the media, advertising, other patients' experiences and their friends. These beliefs may be incorrect or only half true. Sometimes, misconceptions can add to the difficulties of adjusting to kidney failure. For instance, people who believe that nothing is seriously wrong unless they are in pain are not likely to seek help for a condition that has no obvious symptoms, such as high blood pressure.

5. Support. The amount and quality of support available to patients are further influences on how well they cope with kidney failure:

- People who live alone, away from their family and with few friends, tend to adjust poorly to long-term diseases. Other forms of support are particularly important for these people.

- For many people with kidney failure, the immediate family is the main source of psychological support. For others, this role is taken by one or more close friends. Such support is usually a big help to the person. However, it is also true that relatives and friends sometimes undermine effective coping by providing bad examples or poor advice.

- Hospitals do not always provide people with kidney failure with the support they need. Hospitals can

be dull places for patients, and further depress their mood. Unfortunately, at present, very few renal units have a clinical psychologist. However, there is a general recognition of the need to provide patients with psychological support, and some nurses have had special training in counselling.

- For some people, lack of practical support at home may be a problem. Patients may have difficulty getting round the house or doing everyday tasks. Many lack equipment that could help them become more self-sufficient.

- Many support groups have been set up by and for people with kidney failure. These groups can provide emotional and sometimes financial support, as well as information. (See the 'Useful Addresses' section on *page 159*.)

COPING STRATEGIES

People with kidney failure use different strategies to help them cope with this long-term illness. Many kidney patients find the following strategies helpful:

1. Denial. In the early stages, it can be very useful to deny the situation or not to take it seriously. This helps people escape from the feeling of being overwhelmed by the disease. It also allows time to organise other, better ways of dealing with the situation. The belief that a person with kidney failure is still the same as everyone else is a very important element in psychological well-being.

2. Information seeking. People often find it helpful to seek information about their disease and its treatment. Becoming expert in a subject may give you a sense of control over it. It is particularly important that you feel able to ask your doctor or nurse questions, and that you ask them to explain anything they have told you in words that are easy for you to understand. There is also a great deal of other information available, from books and websites. The quality of this information does vary considerably, but all the sources listed on pages 158–163 have been looked at by the authors and have been found to be reliable.

3. Disease management. Many patients gain a sense of control over their disease by becoming involved in its management – including being responsible for tablet taking and perhaps doing their own dialysis. Some people find it helpful to keep their own records (for example, of their blood pressure, creatinine, eGFR, Hb, potassium and phosphate levels). It is a good idea to keep these in a file along with copies of all clinic letters and discharge summaries; notes of appointments at the renal clinic (dated, and with a record of who was seen and what decisions were made); details and dates of any operations or other procedures undergone, together with the names of the surgeon, anaesthetist and any other health professionals involved.

4. Prioritising different activities. Some people with kidney failure, find it can be helpful in the long term to reduce the importance of some of their current activities, such as social drinking or playing contact sports.

5. Goal setting. A very useful coping strategy for many people is to set themselves appropriate goals. These might include, for example, exercising or going out, and trying to maintain regular routines.

6. Thinking positively. One of the problems can often be that bad news travels better than good. Join your local kidney patients' association and talk to people who are managing to maintain a good quality of life on dialysis or with a transplant. What can you learn about coping from them? Kidney failure may change your life, but it doesn't need to devastate it.

KEY FACTS

1 Kidney failure has a major impact on the whole of a patient's life.

2 Psychology is about behaviour and beliefs.

3 People with kidney failure have to cope with extra stresses.

4 Kidney failure and its treatment will affect the lives of those who are closest to you, as well as your own.

5 People diagnosed with kidney failure (in common with people affected by many other serious diseases or trauma) usually go through shock, grief and denial before acceptance.

6 Deciding not to follow the treatment guidelines your doctor has given you is referred to as a 'lack of concordance'. Almost a third of patients choose not to follow an agreed treatment regime at some time or another.

7 Failing to follow your treatment regime can be very dangerous and even cause death – so it is vital you ask your doctor to talk through any aspect of your treatment programme you don't feel happy with or find difficult.

8 Other long-term problems may include anxiety, problems with body image, loss of self-confidence, depression, adapting to changes, and a loss of interest in sex.

9 Kidney failure can sometimes affect a person's ability to concentrate and think clearly. Efficient dialysis helps most people.

10 Many factors affect a person's ability to cope with kidney failure, but there are various coping strategies that different people find useful.

11 Some people prefer not to think about the situation, or refuse to take it seriously (denial). Others may adopt a structured approach, managing their own illness as far as possible, prioritising different activities or goal setting. It is important you follow the approach that works best for you.

16 SEXUAL PROBLEMS

This chapter describes the problems commonly experienced by men and women with kidney failure. It examines the causes of these problems, and makes some suggestions as to what can be done about them.

INTRODUCTION

Although some kidney patients never have sexual problems, many others do. Sometimes, sexual problems start quite early in kidney failure, before dialysis is needed. Patients may then experience an improvement in their sex lives when they start dialysis, although some notice no difference. Other patients with kidney failure develop sexual problems only after they start dialysis (either PD or haemodialysis). A kidney transplant often improves a person's sex life, but problems may continue.

INVESTIGATING SEXUAL PROBLEMS

In the past, many health professionals working with kidney patients have tended to avoid getting involved with their patients' sexual problems. Patients, doctors and nurses have often been embarrassed to discuss the subject. Even now, despite the more general interest in and openness about sexual matters, people with kidney failure may still find that they have to raise the subject first.

As with other aspects of kidney failure, it is not usually a case of just one straightforward problem that can be easily corrected. Often there are several issues to

look at, and patience is required. Nevertheless, treatment is usually successful, provided both partners are keen to have a sex life and are willing to accept help.

ERECTILE DYSFUNCTION (IMPOTENCE)

Men with kidney failure have a variety of sexual problems. These include having sex less often, loss of interest in sex (sometimes called loss of libido), and being unable to ejaculate ('come'). However, the most common sexual problem – and often the most worrying one for a man – is difficulty in getting or keeping a hard penis. This was generally known as 'impotence' but you may well find your doctor uses the term 'erectile dysfunction' or 'ED' instead.

What normally happens first in men with kidney failure is that they become less able to keep an erection for as long as usual, although they are still able to ejaculate. Eventually, many kidney patients lose the ability to get a hard penis at all. Obviously, this can lead to frustration, particularly if the sex drive is unchanged. The situation can be even more upsetting if the man's partner interprets the problem as a loss of interest in her personally.

WHAT CAUSES ERECTILE DYSFUNCTION?

Erectile dysfunction has many possible causes. In most men with kidney failure, sexual problems do not have just one cause, but are usually due to a combination of:

1. Poor blood supply. In order to make the penis hard, extra blood enters the penis and is then prevented from leaving it. Many kidney patients have narrowed blood vessels all over their body, including those vessels that supply the penis. This reduces the blood supply to the penis, and makes it difficult to get an erection. It is not just kidney patients who have this problem. It also occurs as part of the natural ageing process and is more common in older men as well as in men with diabetes.

2. Leaky blood vessels. To keep the penis hard, the extra blood that has entered the penis must stay inside it. In men with kidney failure, the extra blood sometimes leaks back out of the penis, and so the erection is lost.

3. Hormonal disturbances. Hormones are chemical messengers that control many body functions. They are carried around the body in the blood. Some hormones are specifically designed to control sexual urges. The levels of these sex hormones can be either higher or lower than normal in people with kidney failure. In particular, the testicles may produce less of the male sex hormone, testosterone.

4. Nerve damage. The nerves that supply the penis are also involved in getting an erection. When someone has kidney failure, nerve damage may prevent the nerves from working properly.

5. Tablets. Most tablets do not cause erectile dysfunction on their own. However, a few drugs can contribute to sexual problems. The biggest culprits are the blood pressure tablets called beta-blockers, such as atenolol, propranolol, metoprolol and bisoprolol.

6. Tiredness. Tiredness can affect sexual performance. Tiredness in a kidney patient may be caused by anaemia (see Chapter 5), by under-dialysis (see page 14), or by other medical problems, such as heart problems.

7. Psychological problems. When a kidney patient starts dialysis, there are many stresses to deal with (see Chapter 15). Not surprisingly, some patients feel quite depressed. If so, they may not feel like having sex.

8. Relationship difficulties. The illness of one partner naturally causes stresses in a relationship. For instance, household jobs such as decorating or mowing the lawn, which used to be done by the patient, may now have to be done by the partner. This can lead to arguments or resentment on either side of the relationship.

The normal erection process

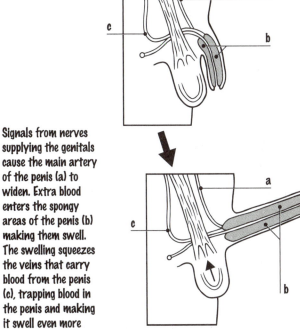

Signals from nerves supplying the genitals cause the main artery of the penis (a) to widen. Extra blood enters the spongy areas of the penis (b) making them swell. The swelling squeezes the veins that carry blood from the penis (c), trapping blood in the penis and making it swell even more

HOW IS ERECTILE DYSFUNCTION INVESTIGATED?

The first and most important step is for the subject to be raised. There is often a lot of unnecessary suffering due either to denial of the problem or to fear of embarrassment. Some kidney doctors and nurses have no experience of treating sexual problems in people with kidney failure, or are embarrassed themselves. If this is the case, patients should ask to see an expert in sexual problems. Sadly, few kidney units have access to such an expert at present.

Once the problem of erectile dysfunction has been recognised, the following should take place:

1. A general health check. This will include an assessment of the distance a person can walk on level ground without having to stop, which is a useful guide to general health.

2. Physical examination. This will include an examination of the genitals. The doctor will also feel for a pulse at various points in the legs. If the pulses are weak, this means that the blood vessels in the legs have narrowed, reducing the blood supply. There will then usually also be narrowing of the blood vessels supplying the penis, reducing its blood supply.

3. Blood tests. In addition to the usual blood tests, there will be tests to measure the blood levels of various hormones. These include testosterone, and also luteinising hormone (LH), follicle-stimulating hormone (FSH) and prolactin. LH and FSH are hormones that regulate the testicles. Prolactin's usual role is to produce milk in females, but it is often present in larger than normal amounts in male dialysis patients with erectile dysfunction.

4. Review of medication. The doctor should review the various tablets that the person is taking. Some types of tablet may contribute to sexual difficulties. Alternative medication is sometimes available.

5. Investigation of psycho-sexual problems. The doctor will ask the patient to consider whether psychological or relationship difficulties may be contributing to the physical problem of erectile dysfunction.

HOW IS ERECTILE DYSFUNCTION TREATED?

The doctor will begin by looking at any more general problems that may be contributing to erectile dysfunction. These may include:

- treating anaemia (see *Chapter 5*);
- increasing the amount of dialysis; and
- changing the patient's tablets.

More specific physical treatments for erectile dysfunction will then be considered. These may include:

- tablets (Viagra and Cialis);
- hormone treatment;
- use of a vacuum device;
- penile injection therapy;
- penile insertion therapy (putting a drug down the penis); and
- penile implants.

In addition to the various physical treatment options (see *below* for more details), patients may be recommended to seek help for emotional problems relating to erectile dysfunction (see *page 121*).

Men who are on dialysis or have a kidney transplant can have treatment for erectile dysfunction free of charge on the NHS. People who are not getting treatment for kidney failure (i.e. dialysis or a transplant) may not be able to get free treatment for erection difficulties. However, if the doctor thinks the problems caused by erectile dysfunction are causing a lot of distress, treatment might be free.

TABLETS (VIAGRA AND CIALIS)

Viagra (sildenafil) is the best known tablet for treating erectile dysfunction. It has had a lot of publicity since it first became available in America in April 1998. It works by opening up the blood vessels in the penis. This causes the man to have an erection.

An early trials of Viagra in kidney patients with erectile dysfunction who also had diabetes showed that the drug worked well in about half of them. However, they did get some side effects from the drug. These were occasional headaches, indigestion and muscle aches. People who have a condition called angina and use GTN (a spray which relieves the pain), and people who have very low blood pressure, should not take Viagra.

During the past few years, Viagra has become the first choice of treatment for kidney patients with erection problems. It works well in around 75% of the dialysis and transplant patients (diabetic or not) who take it. Many patients even say it lasts longer than usual – it can still be effective 'the morning after'!

Another drug, Cialis (tadalafil), has similar effects. Doctors think this may not be suitable for all people with kidney failure. However, other drugs are being developed all the time.

HORMONES

Most male dialysis patients with sexual problems have lowish testosterone levels. This deficiency can be treated by an injection of testosterone every 3–4 weeks, or by using testosterone replacement patches (such as the Andropatch). Although testosterone therapies replace the hormone that is lacking, they are not always very effective in treating impotence. This is probably because impotence in men with kidney failure is not usually due only to low testosterone levels.

Many other hormones are also often found to be at the wrong level, but correcting them rarely makes much difference to sexual difficulties. If the prolactin level is too high, a tablet such as cabergoline or bromocriptine may be given. However, these tablets are not always very successful at making erection problems better.

VACUUM DEVICES

Many kidney patients with erectile dysfunction require therapies which act directly on the penis, helping them to get and keep an erection. One of these is called vacuum tumescence therapy, which uses a mechanical device (such as the ErecAid) to produce a hard penis. Nearly three quarters of the male dialysis patients who use a vacuum device are able to have full penile erections.

To use the vacuum device, the man first inserts his penis into the clear plastic cylinder. He then holds the device against his body so that the chamber is closed with an air-tight seal. Using either a hand- or battery-operated pump, the man then withdraws air from the cylinder to form a vacuum. This causes the penis to enlarge in a way that is similar to a natural erection. However, to maintain the erection, the man must then push a tension ring (resembling an elastic band) from the outside of the cylinder onto the base of the penis. The seal of the vacuum is broken, and the cylinder and pump are removed. With the tension ring in place, the erection can be maintained for up to 30 minutes.

The erections may be longer lasting than natural ones, and do not usually disappear after an orgasm. The most common complaints are mild discomfort and 'timing difficulties' (such as pumping too rapidly with the hand-pump) when the device is first used. Occasionally, harmless, tiny reddish spots (called petechiae) may appear on the penis.

The main advantages of vacuum therapy are that it is safe and non-surgical, can be used as often as desired, and works well for most male dialysis patients. Its suppliers also claim that it may improve blood flow to the penis and result in occasional natural erections.

An ErecAid

1 The man's penis is inserted into the plastic cylinder of the ErecAid. The ErecAid is then held against the body to form an airtight seal

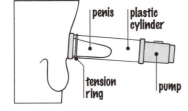

penis | plastic cylinder

tension ring | pump

2 The man uses the pump to withdraw air from the cylinder forming a vacuum. The penis enlarges in a similar way to a natural erection

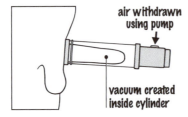

air withdrawn using pump

vacuum created inside cylinder

3 The tension ring is slipped off the ErecAid onto the base of the penis to help maintain the erection, and the ErecAid is then removed

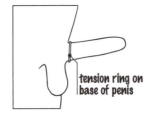

tension ring on base of penis

The disadvantages of vacuum therapy are that it involves a loss of spontaneity in lovemaking, it requires some skill to use, and it can cause mild bruising.

PENILE INJECTION THERAPY

Penile injection therapy is another non-surgical technique used to treat erectile dysfunction. The man injects medication (usually alprostadil) into the base of his penis. This causes the penis to become hard almost immediately. The erection then lasts for 1–2 hours.

The use of the injection is limited to not more than once a day and three times a week. Several clinic visits are usually needed to establish the dose of medication required. The treatment is available on the NHS.

Penile injections have the advantage of not involving surgery. They are also effective in many dialysis patients. The main problems with this technique are pain in the penis, and a condition called priapism, which is an unwanted erection that goes on too long. There may also be bleeding, bruising or scarring (fibrosis) at the injection site. Because of the risk of bleeding, patients on haemodialysis are advised not to have the injection on a dialysis day because of the heparin used during dialysis (see page 75). Another problem is that the penis may become mis-shaped. After a while, some patients get fed up with having these injections, but it is usually possible for them to change to another type of treatment.

PENILE INSERTION (TRANSURETHRAL) THERAPY

Patients who use this treatment have to pass urine beforehand. This makes insertion of the pellet easier (because of the lubrication), and it also helps to dissolve the pellet. Some patients who don't pass much urine may therefore have difficulty using this treatment.

Penile insertion therapy, such as MUSE (Medicated Urethral System for Erection), involves the patient slowly inserting an applicator into the end of his penis. A button on the applicator is then pressed to release a tiny pellet of medication (alprostadil). Once the pellet has been released, the applicator is removed and an erection develops over the next 10–30 minutes.

Penile insertion therapy has been shown to be successful in just over half the men treated in the general population. The most common side effects are penile discomfort or burning, and light-headedness. Female partners have occasionally reported vaginal burning or itching.

Penile insertion therapy is likely to have a slightly higher failure rate than vacuum devices and penile injections. Nevertheless it is a safe, well-tolerated treatment option.

PENILE IMPLANTS

The decision to have a penile implant should be made only after very careful consideration. This surgical treatment for erectile dysfunction is usually effective, but it does have disadvantages (see *below*).

The implant is inserted during an operation performed under a general anaesthetic. There are various different types available. It is usual to have a cylinder implanted in the penis, and connected by a tube to a pump in the scrotum. This pump is connected by another tube to a fluid-containing reservoir in the abdomen (tummy). Squeezing the pump with the fingers causes fluid to pass from the reservoir into the cylinder, so simulating an erection.

The main disadvantage is that the operation to insert the implant alters the penis permanently, ending all hope of natural erections. There is also a risk of infection, and a possibility that the implant will be rejected by the immune system (the body's defence system). Another problem is that an implant can be difficult to conceal.

EMOTIONAL PROBLEMS

Even though the treatments described above usually help to correct erection difficulties, they cannot by themselves restore a sexual relationship.

Sexual problems involve two people, and both partners need to work hard to sort them out. It is very common for people to experience changes in loving relationships after the development of kidney failure. Often, early in kidney disease, one partner becomes the 'carer' and the other adopts the 'sick role'. Later, the improved health of a patient on dialysis, and the desire to restore a sexual relationship, can create new stresses which may take time and patience from both partners to resolve.

Other hidden fears may also be present. For instance, some people may believe that kidney disease could be transferred during sex. This is not true.

Many kidney patients and their partners may want to have counselling, from either a psychologist or a sexual counsellor. This can be very effective, so if you feel it might be helpful in your case, do talk to your GP or renal unit doctor about whether you can be referred to a specialist counsellor.

SEXUAL PROBLEMS FOR WOMEN

Many women who have kidney failure do not have problems with having sex and have happy and fulfilled sex lives. However, there are some specific problems that female patients may experience:

1. Discomfort during sex. Some women do find that sex is sometimes painful. This may be due to a problem with a lack of lubrication (producing juices in the vagina). If this is the case, having more foreplay can help, although using a water-based lubricant (like KY jelly), which is available over the counter from chemists, may be the answer. Another cause of painful sex in women is an infection of the vagina (for example, thrush) or of the womb. If an infection is present, it can easily be treated with antibiotic or antifungal medication.

2. Reduced sex drive. People who need regular dialysis often feel very tired, especially following a session on the haemodialysis machine. However, there are many other reasons that sex drive may be lower than usual, and these include depression, anaemia or a change in roles between partners.

One of the most important things a woman with

kidney failure can do is to make sure her partner knows her feelings for him haven't changed. She can make a point of letting him know he is still valued. Planning something romantic on the days when the tiredness isn't so bad can work wonders.

It is also a good idea to discuss the problems of tiredness and reduced sex drive with the doctor when visiting the kidney unit. The various medications prescribed may make the situation worse for some women.

3. Body image. Some kidney patients have problems and worries with the way they look, especially those on dialysis, because of either the catheter or fistula. This often leads to feeling self-conscious, unattractive and no longer desirable. This in turn can lead to them avoiding sex with their partner. However, it is often only the patient (and not the partner) who feels this way. The truth is that a woman with kidney failure is still the same person with the same lovable characteristics she had before her kidneys failed.

It is very common for patients to lose confidence in themselves and not feel like making love any more. But this can lead either partner to blame themselves, and think that they are no longer attractive. The easiest and often most effective remedy in these situations is to talk to each other. If both partners can reassure each other, and express affection for each other, they will each be well on the way to regaining their confidence.

Many kidney units now have a counsellor who is specially trained to deal with problems such as this. If you are worried and would like professional help, ask your nurse or doctor if you can see a counsellor.

MENSTRUAL PERIODS AND FERTILITY

It is common for the menstrual periods to become irregular when women develop kidney failure. If a woman with kidney failure does not yet need dialysis, she will be less fertile (less likely to become pregnant, even if she is having regular sex) than other women are. However, she should use contraception, as pregnancy is still possible.

In dialysis patients, the periods often stop completely. This means that women on dialysis are not very likely to

RISK OF PROBLEMS DURING PREGNANCY FOR KIDNEY PATIENTS

	Creatinine less than 120 µmol/l (CKF Stage 1)	Creatinine of between 120 and 250 µmol/l (CKF Stage 2)	Creatinine of more than 250 µmol/l (CKF Stages 3–5)
Chance of problems occurring during pregnancy	25%	50%	85%
Chance of the baby being born small		30%	60%
Chance of the baby being born prematurely		55%	70%
Chance of a successful pregnancy	85–95%	60–90%	20–30%

become pregnant. However, again, women should not rely on this as a form of contraception. It is still possible to get pregnant even without having periods.

Treatment with erythropoietin (EPO) has been shown to restore menstrual periods in about 50% of women on dialysis. This is thought to be due to two effects of EPO. It improves disturbed hormone levels, and it treats anaemia (see *Chapter 5*). Treatment with EPO increases a woman's chance of becoming pregnant, so contraception should always be used to avoid an unwanted pregnancy.

PREGNANCY

Many women of child-bearing age who are on dialysis have irregular periods or no periods at all, yet it is still possible for them to become pregnant. However, the success of pregnancy varies widely, depending on the degree of kidney failure. The easiest and most reliable way to calculate the risk to both mother and baby is by estimating the level of kidney function, and this is most easily done by measuring the level of creatinine in the

blood. The table on *page 122* shows the percentage chance of problems occurring, depending on the level of creatinine in the patient's blood when she becomes pregnant. As you can see, women who have a creatinine level of less than 120 µmol/l (micromoles per litre of blood) have a much better chance of a trouble-free pregnancy and having a healthy baby.

If a woman does become pregnant when she already has even mild kidney failure, there is a risk, despite the success of the pregnancy, that her kidney failure will worsen. If you do have kidney failure, but are not yet getting treatment (dialysis or a transplant), it is worth taking this into consideration before trying for a baby. The table below shows the likelihood of kidney damage during pregnancy, depending on the level of creatinine in the patient's blood.

Following a transplant, most women find their periods start again as their hormone levels return to normal, and there is better clearance of the toxins from the body. Oestradiol is one of the hormones controlling a woman's periods, and this is usually restored to normal after a transplant, resulting in a return of normal ovulation (egg

RISKS TO KIDNEY FUNCTION DURING PREGNANCY

	Creatinine less than 120 µmol/l (CKF Stage 1)	Creatinine of between 170 and 220 µmol/l (CKF Stage 2)	Creatinine of more than 220 µmol/l (CKF Stages 3–5)
Chance of losing kidney function	2%	40–65%	75%
Chance of kidney function deteriorating after the birth		20–50%	60%
Chance of severe kidney damage requiring dialysis or transplant		2–33%	40%

production in the ovaries) and periods. Generally speaking, the risks during pregnancy, for the health of the mother and baby, are less for women who have a well-functioning transplant. The table below shows the percentage chance of problems occurring for mothers who have a transplant, depending on the level of creatinine in the blood.

There is also a risk that the patient's transplant kidney may be damaged during the pregnancy; however, this too depends upon the patient's blood creatinine level when she gets pregnant. If the patient's blood creatinine is less than 100 µmol/l, the risk of damaging the transplant kidney is almost nil. However, if the patient's blood creatinine is between 100 and 130 µmol/l during the pregnancy, there is a 15% chance that the transplant will have failed after 8 years. For women whose creatinine is more than 130 µmol/l when they become pregnant, there is a 35% chance that the transplant kidney will have failed after 3 years.

Kidney transplant patients who do get pregnant will be under the care of both the kidney and maternity teams. They will work together with the patient's GP and midwife throughout the pregnancy. It is important to monitor the kidney function and blood pressure during pregnancy. The drugs that transplant patients take to prevent rejection are unlikely to cause any problems during the pregnancy. Even so, it is best to tell your kidney doctor if you are planning to become pregnant, or as soon as you find out.

Once the baby is born, some of the drugs can be passed through breast milk, but many doctors feel that the benefits of breastfeeding the baby outweigh the risks.

Overall, if a woman with kidney failure wants to get pregnant, it is best for her to do so either in the early stages of kidney failure or after she has had a transplant (as long as it is working well). It should be pointed out that the baby is as likely as any other baby to be normal, and will not usually inherit the mother's condition. Nonetheless, any woman with kidney failure who is thinking about having a family should consider all the potential problems and risks, both for herself and for the baby, before going ahead. If she is in any doubt at all

RISK OF PROBLEMS DURING PREGNANCY FOR KIDNEY TRANSPLANT PATIENTS

	Creatinine less than 120 µmol/l (CKF Stage 1)	Creatinine of more than 120 µmol/l (CKF Stages 1–5)
Chance of problems during pregnancy	30%	82%
Chance of a successful pregnancy	97%	75%
Chance of the mother having long-term health problems	7%	27%

about whether to try for a baby, she should speak to the doctors and nurses in the kidney unit. They are there to help people make decisions like this.

If the risks are considered too great, some form of contraception is recommended. The Pill is best avoided in women who have high blood pressure or clotting problems. Other methods of contraception, such as the coil (intra-uterine device) or condoms, can be discussed with the doctor.

It is also a good idea to practise 'safe sex' by using condoms. This will reduce your risk of getting AIDS and other sexually transmitted diseases.

KEY FACTS

1 Sexual difficulties affect the majority of male and female dialysis patients.

2 You may find that doctors and nurses are reluctant to talk about sexual problems, and that it is down to you to raise the subject.

3 Erectile dysfunction (difficulty in getting or keeping a hard penis) is the most common and worrying problem for men with kidney failure.

4 Treatment of erectile dysfunction is usually successful, although you may need to be very patient.

5 Treating anaemia, adjusting the amount of dialysis and changing tablets can all help.

6 Viagra tablets have been shown to be effective in many dialysis patients, as have vacuum devices. Other tablets now available include Cialis.

7 Penile injection therapy may be successful, although there are disadvantages.

8 Penile insertion (transurethral) therapy is slightly less effective than some other treatments. Men must also be able to pass urine before using it.

9 Sex and relationship counselling can be helpful. Talk to your doctor about whether you can be referred for this if you feel you and your partner would benefit.

10 Kidney failure affects women's periods. Pregnancy is less likely, but contraception is still needed.

11 A successful pregnancy is sometimes possible, but there are considerable risks for both mother and baby. It is important to discuss the risks with your doctor, if at all possible, before getting pregnant.

12 If you are a woman with kidney failure, and you want to have a baby, it is best for you to try to get pregnant either in the early stages of kidney failure or after a transplant, as long as the transplant is working well.

17 DEATH AND DYING

This chapter explores some of those difficult issues around the subject of death and dying. The intention is to give readers the information necessary to make choices at the appropriate time – the best choices for them and those they love.

INTRODUCTION

Death is a subject seldom discussed openly with patients in a dialysis unit. Dialysis and kidney transplants represent, after all, the success of our knowledge and skill in conquering a previously fatal illness. These treatments are *all about life*. Yet nobody can attend a kidney unit without the realisation that death is always close at hand. In a large dialysis centre, a week rarely passes without someone dying. Units are close communities, where patients know many of those attending as friends. Each of them will be aware, therefore, of a succession of losses, reminding them of the fragility of their own lives.

People with kidney failure live with the knowledge that they have a shorter life expectancy than the rest of the population (as can be seen from the tables in *Chapter 18*). The cause of death is not usually kidney failure, with the exception of one important group – those who choose not to receive dialysis. We feel it is right, therefore, to include a chapter in this book, acknowledging the fact that what doctors can provide is far from perfect.

There is no doubt that life on dialysis can be full, rewarding and worthwhile for many people. However, there are some who feel either that they would not wish to live with the limitations imposed by treatment, or that

they have done so long enough. When the need for dialysis approaches, those who are already elderly, or whose lives are seriously restricted by other illnesses, may decide that they would rather allow nature to 'take its course' – even though this means they will die. Some, therefore, choose not to start dialysis treatment. There are others, who may have dialysed for many years, becoming more frail or disabled as time goes on, who decide that the time has come to stop treatment and die with dignity.

It is important for patients and their families to understand that *dialysis is not compulsory*. If you do not wish to receive treatment, or decide that you wish to stop dialysis, you should discuss this with the staff at your renal unit. Remember that *only you* can judge whether your quality of life is acceptable. You may be frail or elderly, severely disabled or restricted, yet satisfied that life is still worthwhile. If this is the case, starting or continuing dialysis is 'right for you'. You may, on the other hand, appear to be doing quite well in the opinion of others – yet, in your eyes, life is intolerable. It is *your* point of view that counts.

Most units have a sympathetic attitude and will offer you all the information and support you need in taking this decision.

DEATH FROM KIDNEY FAILURE

Patients are often afraid to ask renal unit staff, whose lives are devoted to maintaining life against the odds, what it is like to die from kidney failure. While every death is different (just as every life is different), it can be said with some confidence that it is, in general, 'not a bad way to go'. The problems that occur in the final days of death from kidney failure vary from person to person. The symptoms that may need to be controlled include feeling sick (nausea), muscle twitching and breathlessness. Sometimes there is some agitation and confusion. Pain is not usually a serious problem.

Nausea can be caused by the waste products, usually removed by normal kidneys, building up in the blood. There are several drugs available that can be used to reduce or prevent nausea. Breathlessness may be due to fluid overload. Both drugs and suction treatment can be used to keep the lungs clear to reduce breathlessness, while carefully administered drug treatment can keep the patient comfortable and free from distress. Most of the drugs used for nausea, breathlessness or agitation (e.g. morphine and similar drugs) cause some degree of sedation, leading to drowsiness.

Patients and families usually want to know how long a person can survive with untreated ERF. This too is variable, depending on the extent to which their old kidneys are working – and therefore the amount of urine that they pass. The kidneys may be able to get rid of some excess fluid, but unable to process waste products such as creatinine and urea, or salts such as potassium. It is the build-up of these substances in the blood (especially the potassium) that usually leads to death.

On average, patients who are passing reasonable amounts of urine (say over 1 litre per day) can survive for about 2–6 weeks. If little or no urine is passed, they may survive for 10–14 days. During this period, they generally become increasingly weak and drowsy, sleep more and more, and finally become unconscious. Then they will pass away peacefully.

WHERE SHOULD THIS PERIOD BE SPENT?

This is very much up to the individual and family. If a patient wishes to be at home, specialist nursing can be arranged through the GP. It is very important for some people to feel they are in familiar surroundings, with family members and pets around them. Whenever this is the case, people with ERF should receive every support to spend their last days at home.

Some hospices (which mainly deal with patients dying from cancer) will admit kidney patients who have decided to stop dialysis or not to start it in the first place. Hospice care and support of the dying is particularly sympathetic, taking into account the needs and feelings of both patient and family.

Most kidney units are experienced in the care of dying patients, who are usually nursed in a side ward, offering quiet and privacy. It is usual for relatives to be allowed to stay with the patient all the time. Some kidney units offer accommodation in a 'relatives' room'. One of the benefits of remaining in hospital is that, if the person has a change of heart and decides to go for dialysis after all, the facilities are close at hand.

THE DECISION NOT TO START DIALYSIS TREATMENT

If a person attending a pre-dialysis clinic tells the kidney consultant that, when the need arises, he or she does not want dialysis treatment, it is important that this decision is made with full knowledge – it is an 'informed' choice.

In the first place, the patient needs to ask the doctor, quite directly, about the likely outcome – i.e. how long they might expect to live both with and without dialysis, and also what can be done to make their last days comfortable if they choose not to dialyse. This information is essential for making a rational decision. It may be that, with dietary care and medication, a person would live for some months, free of frequent hospital visits or preparations for treatment such as access surgery. This is particularly true in the case of very elderly people, leading an inactive life.

We do not know that dialysis necessarily prolongs the life of all very frail elderly people (especially those over, say, 80 years of age). This does not mean they will not be offered the treatment. If dialysis does prolong life a little, then the quality of that life could be poorer than it would have been had dialysis not been started. One research study looking at frail elderly patients found that the average length of survival on dialysis was 8 months, whereas a similar population without dialysis could expect to live for 6 months. In other words, dialysis prolonged the patients' lives by 2 months. In addition to this, most of the patients who did receive dialysis spent a high proportion of their 8 months in hospital, and many died in hospital. The majority of the other (non-dialysis group) on the other hand, died at home.

It is important to be aware too that it is impossible to know exactly what life on dialysis is like unless one has experienced it. Even talking to others receiving treatment does not give the full picture, as everyone is different. Sometimes, patients agree to treatment reluctantly, only to find that it is not nearly as bad as they had imagined it would be. Others tell us that, on the contrary, they had expected it to be much easier to cope with, or that they had hoped to feel far better on treatment than they actually do.

TRIALS OF DIALYSIS

To discover what life on dialysis is like, some patients opt for a 'trial of dialysis', lasting a few weeks or months. This allows them to discover both the good and bad sides of life on dialysis, and to decide whether the benefits outweigh the drawbacks.

In some cases, a short period of treatment may be undertaken in order to give patients time to settle their affairs, or resolve conflicting feelings in the family.

These are not uncommon during the heightened emotional tension surrounding such a decision. Others need time to allow visits from family members living abroad, and to say goodbye. Everything should be done that will allow the patient peace of mind. Relatives, too, need a sense of resolution, free from unnecessary guilt and regret.

CHOOSING THE LESSER OF TWO EVILS

There may be good medical reasons to decide not to dialyse, without even considering a trial of treatment. If a patient with kidney failure is already suffering from another terminal illness, for example an inoperable cancer, a progressive neurological or vascular disease (such as recurrent strokes) or severe heart failure, it can be a blessing in disguise to be offered the opportunity of refusing dialysis. This can allow a dignified death, in less distressing circumstances than might otherwise apply. Those who need dialysis to stay alive have a control over the time and manner of their death that is denied to most other people.

THOSE WHO CANNOT MAKE AN INFORMED CHOICE

So far, we have only considered those people who are in a position to make an informed choice. Sadly, some patients may have a condition or illness that makes it impossible for them to choose what they wish to do. Those with advanced dementia (with Alzheimer's disease, for example) or severe learning difficulties may not be able to understand the implications of the decision. They might, in addition, be unable to understand the necessity of attending for dialysis, or of observing diet and fluid restriction – and would, in all probability, find the treatment very hard to tolerate. Each case needs to be considered on its merits, with the patient's best interests always in mind.

People who have had a stroke causing irreversible brain damage, or an illness or injury that makes them drowsy or semi-conscious all the time, cannot express an opinion about their wishes. In these cases, it is much more difficult for the doctors to know how to act for the best – i.e. in the patient's best interests. It can be helpful, especially for the relatives, if people with kidney failure make their wishes known at a time when they are able to decide for themselves.

If you feel that there are circumstances in which you would not wish to be kept alive by dialysis, you can confirm this in writing, and ask for the document to be kept in your medical notes. While this document, sometimes called a 'Living Will' or an 'Advanced Directive', has no legal status, it is valuable in giving a guide to your doctor and next of kin, and in reducing any feelings of guilt your family may experience after your death.

Most kidney consultants will discuss all the options with the family, the patient's GP, the multidisciplinary team in the unit, and any others close to the patient. The consultant has the final responsibility for deciding what is in the best interests of the patient, having taken everyone's views into consideration.

THE DECISION TO STOP DIALYSIS

Withdrawal from dialysis is not an uncommon cause of death in long-standing dialysis patients, particularly those who are elderly. In fact, up to 20% of patients die in this way.

For some people, dialysis can become like a treadmill, or a conveyor belt, on which they feel as if they are trapped. The truth is that nobody can force a patient to attend for dialysis. To dialyse somebody against his or her will is legally an 'assault'.

Sometimes, the very knowledge that they are able to stop when they wish is enough to give individuals the will to carry on for the present.

Patients sometimes fear that they are 'letting down' the staff of the kidney unit by wanting to stop treatment. It can seem like ingratitude, or a rejection of the care they have been given. While staff will be sad, they may also be relieved, having been aware of the person's distress. They should, in any case, respect the patient's decision. Nobody can know fully what life is like for another person.

There are many reasons why this decision may be taken. Probably the most common is that the patient suffers a medical setback, often unrelated to the kidneys, such as a stroke. In patients with diabetes, needing to have a limb amputated would be such a setback. It would inevitably result in further disability and limitation, which the patient might regard as just too much to cope with. Life on dialysis may have been tolerable, but the additional problem may remove what quality remained in the patient's life. Loss of independence is often the deciding factor.

The second most common reason for withdrawal is the gradual deterioration caused by ageing and the complications of many years of dialysis. The patient may have considerable pain and restriction from renal bone disease, or problems with blood circulation from narrowing of the arteries.

Dialysis access may have become difficult over the years, leading to frequent hospital admissions. Older patients may also have been bereaved due to the death of their spouse, resulting in less motivation to carry on for the sake of others. Whatever the reasons, the person may feel that it is no longer worth the struggle to continue.

If a patient asks renal unit staff to discontinue dialysis, the subject should be gently explored, to see whether there is anything that can be done to improve the situation. In some people, the request to withdraw is a cry for help, or an expression of a state of depression that could be helped either by sympathetic counselling or by medication. In some cases, patients may be asked to talk things over with a counsellor, psychologist or psychiatrist, to discover whether this is the case. Stopping dialysis is a decision that should not be rushed, but properly considered. Some patients wish to stop, but find their families become distressed by the suggestion. It is important that the feelings of the others who are involved are considered and explored, but the final decision should be the patient's alone.

WITHDRAWING FROM TREATMENT AFTER TRANSPLANT

While successful transplantation offers the best possible quality of life for a patient with kidney failure, it is not without risks. The powerful drugs used to prevent rejection can lead to infections, skin cancers and, in a minority of cases, more serious cancers, especially lymphoma. There is growing concern that newer, stronger drugs which are better at preventing rejection may also be 'better' at stopping the immune system from preventing cancer. It is possible, therefore, that cancer is becoming more common in patients on these drugs. Patients need to be aware of the risks as well as the benefits of transplantation and to discuss their concerns with their consultant. (More information about the risks of transplantation can be found in *Chapter 13*.)

One of the treatments for some serious types of cancer (including lymphoma) is to stop (or reduce the doses of) the immuno-suppressant drugs. In this case, the kidney may be rejected and the patient will need to go back onto dialysis. If the cancer is so advanced that no measures will prevent it, the patient is left with a bleak decision. Life might be prolonged for a short time by stopping the immuno-suppressant drugs and returning to dialysis. But this involves more time spent in hospital when time is short in any case. The advantage of being on dialysis is that the patient can choose when they've had enough, and decide to withdraw. Some patients, however, feel it is preferable to continue the immuno-suppressant drugs and maintain the kidney, but allow the cancer to take a quicker course. Should you be unlucky enough to find yourself in this situation, your doctors should be able to guide you as to the best decision in your particular case.

Other patients, who have had a long period of successful transplantation, develop an incurable condition not related to the drugs they are taking. These patients have a range of options which their doctor should discuss with them. One option might be to stop taking their immuno-suppressant medicine and allow the kidney to reject (and fail). Then they could die from kidney failure without dialysis, if the death from kidney failure is 'better' than it would have been from their new incurable disease. Or, if the incurable disease is killing them slowly, they might decide not to have dialysis when their transplant 'naturally' fails at a later date.

There is another group of patients, often elderly ones, who are not dying of an incurable disease. But the build-up of serious although non-fatal complications of kidney failure (such as bone pain or 'access' problems) is becoming too much for them. So they can 'take the opportunity' of their transplant's 'natural failure' to allow themselves to die, rather than suffer a new period of dialysis – especially when they know they are now unfit to have another transplant and would otherwise have to have dialysis until they die anyway.

SPIRITUAL CONCERNS

Those who do not wish to receive dialysis or stop treatment after receiving it sometimes express concerns that this is the equivalent of suicide, and therefore against the teachings of most major religions. The same views might also be expressed by patients who allow their transplants to fail then refuse dialysis. However, leaders from a number of different faiths have considered the case of the kidney patient who wishes to withdraw from treatment, and none has concluded that such withdrawal is either suicidal or sinful. The basis for this is that, but for an artificial and highly technological treatment, the patient would have died naturally in the first place. One could see this as the original decree of fate, nature or the Deity. As a result of human intervention, the patient has lived beyond his or her natural term. To give up dialysis or stop taking immuno-suppressant drugs is simply to cease prolonging life unnaturally in someone whose body is not capable of sustaining itself.

Any patient, or relative of a patient, who has any concerns, or needs spiritual support, should talk to his or her priest or religious leader. Many hospitals now have a chaplaincy service, with leaders from all the major faiths available to give support and advice.

KEY FACTS

1 Dialysis is not compulsory. A trial of treatment may be a sensible option, while you are making up your mind.

2 Withdrawal from dialysis is not uncommon, especially in older patients.

3 The reason for withdrawal is usually a medical event unrelated to the kidneys – such as a stroke or cancer.

4 The decision should not be rushed, allowing time for others to come to terms with the situation.

5 Death from renal failure need not be distressing, if well managed. It should take place where the patient feels most comfortable.

6 The wish to stop dialysis may be due to depression, or a cry for help, needing action to improve some intolerable situation.

7 Kidney patients have greater control in ensuring a dignified death than most other people.

8 Where a patient is not capable of an informed choice, the consultant has the final responsibility, after discussion with everybody concerned.

9 Transplant patients can decide to stop their immuno-suppressant drugs, to make them reject and lose the kidney, and then not have dialysis. In this way, they can allow themselves to die of kidney failure.

10 Refusing dialysis, or deliberately allowing a transplant to fail, is not suicide. A patient who wishes to take this route should not be made to feel guilty.

11 If religion is important to a patient, it is a good idea for them to discuss these issues with a priest or other religious leader – either from their own community or from the hospital.

18 STATISTICS AND OUTCOMES

This chapter looks at the effect of kidney failure on a patient's life expectancy. It goes on to consider the levels of care available to kidney patients in the UK and in other countries, and how this is likely to change in the future.

INTRODUCTION

The number of patients being treated for kidney failure in the UK has increased in recent years. Without dialysis or a transplant anyone with established renal failure (ERF) will die within a few weeks. With successful treatment, some people with ERF can expect to live for many years. However, it is still true that not enough patients in the UK are getting the treatment they need. This is the case for both dialysis and transplantation, and the latter part of the chapter considers some of the reasons why this might be.

SURVIVAL WITH KIDNEY FAILURE

Kidney function is essential for life. Once a person's own kidneys fail, some form of treatment is necessary if they are to go on living. Currently there are two forms of treatment – dialysis (in which the kidney function is taken over by artificial means), and transplant (in which another person's kidney is used instead). Successful treatment – by dialysis or a transplant – now gives people with kidney failure a new lease of life, sometimes for many years. But how many years?

PERCENTAGE SURVIVAL FOR PEOPLE ON DIALYSIS, ACCORDING TO AGE AT START OF DIALYSIS

Age	1 year	5 years	10 years
20–29	94	82	69
30–39	92	70	51
40–49	89	60	38
50–59	86	47	20
60–64	81	36	10
65–69	77	27	6
70–79	70	18	3
80+	59	8	1
All	**78**	**38**	**20**

(Source: USRDS – United States Renal Data System – 2005)

The 'Survival on Dialysis according to age' table on the left shows the percentage chances of still being alive one, five and ten years after the start of dialysis. People who start dialysis when they are young clearly have a better chance of surviving for longer than people who start dialysis later in life. Perhaps this point is not surprising, given that older people are more likely to die than younger people when they do not have kidney failure. However, people on dialysis have much less chance of surviving for 5 years than healthy people in the same age group.

This data is worrying, especially when you look at patients in middle-life. As you can see, people in the 40–60 age group have only about a 50% chance of being alive after 5 years of the diagnosis of ERF. A fair proportion (say 20–30%) of the younger patients also don't make it to 5 years.

Conversely, you could argue that the data for the elderly (70–79 years) is not too bad, with 70% surviving one year, and 20% 5 years. People in this age group may well consider this gain in life worth having. Similarly, recent UK data (collected by the Renal Registry in 2005) is relatively optimistic for the older age groups, suggesting that people over 75 years live for 21 months on average after starting dialysis.

Another way of looking at survival is to look at the average number of years a person is likely to live, after the start of dialysis, and comparing it to the life expectancy of the population as a whole. This is summarised in the table on the right.

Again, the data is worrying. The table indicates that a 35–39 year old on dialysis has a life expectancy of 9 years, compared to 42 years for someone from the general population (most people live to about 80 these days).

The age group most likely to develop ERF is the 60–64-year-old age group, among whom the average survival time is just over 4 years.

In other words, ERF has a major effect on life

LIFE EXPECTANCY (IN YEARS) AT DIFFERENT AGE GROUPS

Age group	Population as a whole	Dialysis patients
20–24	56.3	13.9
25–29	51.1	12
30–34	46.8	10.5
35–39	42.1	9
40–44	37.5	7.8
45–49	33	6.8
50–54	28.6	5.9
55–59	24.4	5
60–64	20.4	4.3
65–69	16.8	3.7
70–74	13.4	3.1
75–79	10.4	2.6
80–84	7.8	2.2
85+	4.3	1.8

(Source: USRDS 2005)

expectancy, even in the young, reducing it fourfold. In fact, if you look through the age groups, there is about a fourfold difference in life expectancy. But an older patient may be very grateful for the two years (on average) of life they may gain, so there is every reason to offer dialysis to the older person.

These figures include all patients, whatever the cause of their kidney failure, but the life expectancy will be higher in patients with a 'good-outlook' cause of ERF,

133

and lower in a 'bad-outlook' cause. For example, the average survival for patients with diabetes is 3 years, it is 18 months for patients with myeloma and one year for patients with amyloidosis. So, you can see that kidney failure, of whatever cause, is likely to reduce the patient's natural life-span dramatically. The latest figures from the United States suggest that 22% of patients die during the first year they are on dialysis and 8% within the first 3 months.

WHY DO PEOPLE WITH KIDNEY FAILURE DIE?

Although people with kidney failure have a lower than average life expectancy, once they start treatment (by either dialysis or a transplant) they are more likely to die from something other than kidney disease. The most common reason that people with kidney failure die is because they have heart disease as well.

Perhaps this is not surprising as, in most developed countries, a large number of people in the population as a whole (29%) die of heart disease. Cancer (23%) and strokes (7%) are the next most common causes of death in developed countries. The death rate from stroke is about the same in patients with kidney failure when compared to the general population but there are fewer deaths from cancer. There are also additional causes of death among kidney patients. For example, 18% of UK patients with advanced kidney failure die because they choose to stop dialysis. This and the surrounding issues are discussed fully in Chapter 17.

Also many people with kidney failure die of infections (16% of patients in the UK). Dialysis patients may be prone to peritonitis or infections of access sites (see pages 64–5; 75–6). In transplant patients, infections occur because the patient is taking immuno-suppressant drugs (see page 98) to prevent rejection of the kidney.

Meanwhile, common sense tells us that the general state of a patient's health will also have a bearing on how long that person will live. Everyone, whether or not they have kidney failure, will be at greater risk of dying early if they have had a heart attack or stroke, peripheral vascular disease (narrowing of the arteries to the legs), serious cancers (including myeloma and amyloidosis), and diabetes. If someone with kidney failure has none of these conditions, they have a good chance of long-term survival, either on dialysis or with a transplant.

People are more likely to die from the complications of kidney failure, especially those affecting the heart, than from the kidney failure itself. It seems that permanent damage to the heart often occurs early in kidney failure, before dialysis or a transplant is needed. This damage is probably due to several factors, including

THE MOST COMMON CAUSES OF DEATH IN PEOPLE WITH AND WITHOUT KIDNEY FAILURE

	ERF	Population as a whole
Heart disease	29%	29%
Treatment stopped	18%	?
Infections	16%	<5%
Cancer	10%	23%
Strokes	9%	7%
Others, or uncertain	18%	26%
COPD	?	5%
Accidents/suicide	?	<5%

Source: Renal Registry (2003) and National (USA) Vital Statistics Report (October 2004)

high blood pressure, anaemia and fluid overload. It is also possible that the wastes that build up in the blood in people with kidney failure have a directly toxic effect on the heart. Neither dialysis nor a transplant can do anything to repair an already damaged heart.

INDIVIDUALS NOT STATISTICS

Although statistics can give an indication of the average survival chances of different groups of patients treated for kidney failure, they cannot predict what will happen to any one person. People with kidney failure are

A COMPARISON OF THE NUMBER OF PEOPLE NEWLY DIAGNOSED WITH KIDNEY FAILURE AND RECEIVING TREATMENT IN SEVERAL COUNTRIES (PMP)

Country	2000	2001	2002	2003	% with diabetes
Taiwan	323	357	365		35
USA	325	328	336		44
Japan	252	252	262	265	41
Germany	175	184	174	186	36
Belgium (Dutch-speaking)			170		17
Greece	157	164	165		27
Czech Republic	151	163	157		35
Canada	143	152	154		34
Italy	131	136	142		16
Austria	133	136	132	141	33
Hungary	129	130		139	25
Uruguay	121	124		136	20
Denmark			130	129	22
Spain	132	127	126		22
Turkey	115	141	122		23
Sweden	126	124	125	121	24
New Zealand	110	119	115	112	40
UK	**89**	**95**	**101**	**103**	**18**
Netherlands	93	101	100	101	16
Poland	68	84	99		24
Bosnia and Herzegovina			77	95	
Australia	92	97	94	98	26
Norway	89	95	92	95	16
Finland	90	91	94	93	39

(adapted from *Renal Registry Report 2004*)

individuals not statistics. Even if you belong to a group of patients whose overall chance of survival is poor, you as an individual may still survive for many years. Your survival odds are obviously better if you belong to one of the groups with the best chances of survival.

HOW GOOD ARE THE SERVICES AROUND THE WORLD?

Survival is affected by two things – the severity of a person's disease and the treatment services that are available. While dialysis and transplantation can make an enormous difference to a person's life expectancy, the availability of these treatments does vary from one country to another. One way of assessing how good the services for kidney patients are, is to make comparisons with the services available in other countries.

In order to make useful comparisons about what treatment is available to kidney patients in different countries, it is necessary to take population size into account. This is done by dividing yearly totals from a particular country by the number of millions of people in that country's population. This provides us with tables of comparable figures expressed as numbers per million population (pmp).

The table on page 135 shows the numbers of people diagnosed with kidney failure and starting treatment (by either dialysis or transplant) over several years in different countries, together with the percentage of these who also have diabetes.

In health care, as in football, some countries are clearly better than others. If all football teams were equally good, all teams would gain the same number of points each year – and all would come 'equal top'. Every world cup match would end in a draw. However, not everyone can be top all or even some of the time, and there may be a number of reasons why any country holds the position it does.

One possible explanation is that people from different countries are not similar – that people who live in the UK are not genetically predisposed to developing kidney failure, while Taiwanese and North Americans are. The table shows that Taiwan and the United States have three times as many people per million population with ERF, than the UK. Part of the difference may be explained by the one group of people who are considerably more likely to develop kidney failure than others – i.e. those with diabetes. To account for this, the table has a separate column showing the numbers of people with diabetes. However, this cannot account for all of the difference, as there are other countries (e.g. New Zealand and Finland) with equally high rates of diabetes.

Another reason for the variation in numbers of people being treated is that some countries are better than others at identifying and providing treatment for people who develop kidney failure.

The fact that countries such as Taiwan and the USA have much higher numbers of patients on dialysis than the UK suggests that the UK is failing to treat large numbers of people who develop kidney failure. This is all the more worrying when it is remembered that many people with ERF die within a few weeks unless they are treated by dialysis or a transplant.

Fortunately for kidney patients in the UK, the rate at which patients are starting dialysis is improving (as you can see if you read across the UK row, on the table), but the rate of improvement is still too slow.

THE 'POSTCODE LOTTERY' IN THE UK

The lack of new patients starting dialysis in the UK is a concern. But probably a more major concern is that there are massive differences *within* the UK.

According to the 2004 Renal Registry Report, in 2003, there was a very wide variation in the numbers of new patients starting dialysis around the country –

with the lowest (14 per million per year, in Blaenau Gwent) and highest (231, in Gwynedd) rates both in Wales!

You would imagine, with the high prevalence of diabetes and high blood pressure amongst Blacks and Asians, that units with higher acceptance rates would have relatively high ethnic minority populations. But there is no clear relationship between acceptance rates and the proportion of population from ethnic minorities. In other words, it is not just that busiest units have the greatest numbers of Blacks and Asians in the local population.

Some areas of the UK treat more patients than others – it's as simple as that. Indeed, it is worrying that some areas with large ethnic minorities *don't* have the highest acceptance rates in to dialysis.

RATE OF TRANSPLANTATION

A way of assessing how well different countries are meeting the need for treatment for kidney failure is to compare the number of kidney patients with a functioning transplant. Like the rate for dialysis (see page 135), the rate of kidney transplantation should be similar in all countries. Again, it is easy to see from the table on this page that this is far from being the case. Some countries perform many more kidney transplants than others.

Norway and Spain are the 'transplant kings' of this group of countries. They achieve good results in two different ways. Norway makes sure that all potential living donors are informed about the possibility of helping their loved one. And indeed, they find if they do this, many more do come forward to donate. Spain, on the other hand, emphasises cadaveric transplantation. One way they do this is to have transplant co-ordinators in every main hospital in the land, so that all potential donors are assessed.

Also, when compared to other countries the rates of

NUMBER OF PATIENTS (PMP) WITH A FUNCTIONING TRANSPLANT, IN VARIOUS COUNTRIES

Country	PMP	Country	PMP
Norway	436.9	New Zealand	264.7
Spain	408.5	Czech Republic	240.0
Austria	407.4	Germany	230.2
Sweden	377.6	Hungary	153.8
USA	375.4	Greece	139.4
Finland	353.2	Chile	126.9
Netherlands	317.2	Uruguay	104.9
UK	**290.0**	Poland	97.9
Canada	289.8	Bulgaria	43.4
Australia	273.3	Russia	17.1

(Source: *Renal Registry 2003*)

new transplant pmp in the UK (18.5 cadaveric, 7.2 for living, in 2004–5) is not great either. The Scandinavian countries, in the same time period, had a cadaveric rate of 29.7 pmp and living rate of 12.1 pmp (see the website www.scandiatransplant.org).

As can be seen from this information, the UK's performance in terms of transplantation is mediocre, at best. What is more worrying is that the number of new transplants done in the UK is *decreasing*. In 2004–5, 1307 cadaveric transplants (18.5 pmp) were carried out; compared to 1388 in 2003–4, according to figures on the UK Transplant website (see page 162 for address). Not surprisingly this is failing to keep up with the demand for transplantation, which is *increasing*; from 5074 in 2003–4 to 5425 people waiting in 2004–05.

Unfortunately the rise in the number of living donor transplants performed is lagging behind this; 461 such operations were performed in 2003–04 and 475 (7.2 pmp) in 2004–5.

There is also a wide variation in transplantation services. In 2004–5, in the UK, the number of new heart-beating cadaveric transplants (pmp) was 18.5, with a very wide range from 12.3 (Nottingham) to 28.1 (Cardiff). There was an even greater range in the numbers of new living transplants, from 2.2 pmp (Sheffield) to 23.5 pmp (Coventry); with an average of 7.2 pmp (see the table on *page 141*). So you may be more or less likely to get a transplant, especially a living transplant, according to where you live.

This data comes from UK Transplant, which coordinates transplantation in the UK. You may well find their website helpful – the details are given on *page 162.*

In the next chapter, we look at what policies are being put in place to make sure that good care is shared out fairly around the country. We also look at ways in which people with kidney failure can take control of their own care, and their own lives.

KEY FACTS

1 Without dialysis or a transplant, people die within a few weeks of developing ERF. Successful treatment (by dialysis or a transplant) can prolong life for many years.

2 Even with treatment survival is poor, with about 80% surviving one year, 40% surviving 5 years, and 20% surviving 10 years.

3 Having ERF will shorten a patient's life fourfold. For example, someone aged between 35 and 39 can expect to live a further 9 years compared to 42 years of additional life expectancy for the general, healthy population.

4 Average survival chances for people on dialysis (or after a transplant) are affected by age, the underlying cause of kidney failure and various other medical factors.

5 People with kidney failure are individuals not statistics. Doctors cannot predict for sure what will happen to any one person and that includes you.

6 Some countries treat a far higher proportion of their people who develop kidney failure than do others.

7 The number of people per million population in the UK who are having treatment for kidney failure is much lower than it should be.

8 There is a serious shortfall in the provision of treatment – both dialysis and transplantation – for kidney failure throughout the UK.

9 The UK still suffers from a "postcode lottery" – i.e. you may be more likely to get dialysis and a transplant according to where you live in the UK.

19 NEW DEVELOPMENTS AND CHOICE

The final chapter of this book looks at the developments in the delivery of care to patients with kidney failure throughout the UK. In particular, it considers the recommendations of the new National Service Frameworks and factors that affect patients' choice.

INTRODUCTION

The figures given in the previous chapter show UK services for kidney patients as ranking well behind those of many other countries in the developed world. There are a number of reasons why this could be the case. Two factors are particularly important: there are too few renal units and too few kidney transplants being carried out.

THE NUMBER OF RENAL UNITS

One reason why the provision of treatment for kidney failure in the UK is so low is because this country has relatively few renal units (and therefore relatively few specialist kidney doctors, nurses and other specialist health care workers). This has an impact on the number of patients that can be treated and the number of new patients that are referred for treatment.

In 2000, as part of the NHS Plan, the government announced substantial funding for Renal Services in the UK. They promised that by 2004 there would be 450 new haemodialysis stations available to treat up to 1850 extra patients. To finance this expansion, they invested £18 million in renal services during 2001–2003. Despite this extra money, Renal Services still don't

appear to be able to keep up with demand. The main problem is that kidney failure is relatively expensive to treat. Although it only affects about 0.05% of the UK population, 1.5% of the healthcare budget is spent on treating kidney failure. It is obvious therefore that other ways need to be found to increase the number of patients that can be treated in the UK.

THE NUMBER OF KIDNEY TRANSPLANTS

The other reason for the relatively low treatment rates for kidney failure in the UK could be because there are not enough transplant operations performed to keep up with demand. There are a number of possible sources of kidneys for transplantation – cadaver, living donor and non-heart beating. The most common source of kidneys is cadaveric. However, over recent years, improvements in road safety, seat belt laws and better health care have meant that the number of kidneys that become available for transplantation has decreased. The situation would be improved if more people registered their willingness to donate their organs for transplantation and discussed their wishes with their next of kin.

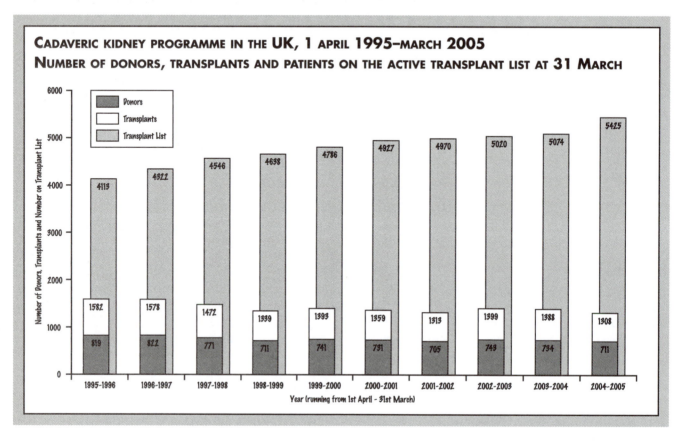

CADAVERIC KIDNEY PROGRAMME IN THE UK, 1 APRIL 1995–MARCH 2005
NUMBER OF DONORS, TRANSPLANTS AND PATIENTS ON THE ACTIVE TRANSPLANT LIST AT 31 MARCH

Even more important is the lack of beds in Intensive Care Units (ICUs) in the UK. If a patient becomes brain dead, and therefore a potential ('heart-beating') kidney donor, that person needs to be kept on a life-support machine to preserve their organs (including their kidneys) until an operation can be performed to remove them. When ICU beds are in short supply, patients who have a chance of recovery must be given priority over patients who are already brain dead. Inevitably, many potential cadaveric organs are lost in this way. Also, relatively few units have a 'non-heart beating' donor programme (see Chapter 12 on Living donor transplants).

As fewer cadaveric transplants are being done, it would make most sense to increase the number of living related (and unrelated) donor transplants, especially as this is the best and cheapest treatment for ERF.

One possible reason why a patient may not be given a living related transplant is that they have no medically suitable donors among their family members. In fact, medical unsuitability among family members is relatively uncommon.

Carrying out a living related or unrelated transplant requires a lot of preparation work by renal doctors, nurses and transplant co-ordinators. Not all renal units in the UK put much time and effort into such work, finding it generally 'easier' (less work) to put patients on the 'normal' (cadaveric) transplant waiting list. Also carrying out transplants from living people means that doctors and nurses are more likely to have to confront 'difficult' issues with patients and their relatives. Perhaps some prefer to avoid this altogether.

The low rate of transplantation from living donors that we have seen across the UK so far, is partly the fault of the doctors and nurses who don't always tell patients and their relatives, partners and friends about the full range of possibilities. If potential donors are not told that kidney donation is a possibility, and are not gently encouraged to come forward, they are unlikely to do so. But donating a kidney to a friend or family member can be more complicated than you think, in all sorts of ways. This will be particularly true if your relationship is not an easy one to start with.

You can see from the table below that there are vast differences in the number of living transplants done throughout the UK. For example, if you are living in

NUMBER OF ADULT LIVING DONOR KIDNEY TRANSPLANTS PERFORMED IN 2004/5

Transplant Centre	Related donor	Unrelated donor	Total	Per million population
Belfast	7	1	8	4.7
Birmingham	25	8	33	7.4
Bristol	12	12	24	12.2
Cambridge	7	6	13	5.2
Cardiff	17	1	18	8
Coventry	14	5	19	23.5
Edinburgh	10	5	15	6.3
Glasgow	11	2	13	4.9
Leeds	20	7	27	7.3
Leicester	17	9	26	12.3
Liverpool	20	5	25	7.7
Manchester	19	4	23	5.8
Newcastle	11	2	13	4.6
North Thames	51	19	70	9.6
Nottingham	9	3	12	8.7
Oxford	12	5	17	5.7
Plymouth	5	0	5	2.8
Portsmouth	9	2	11	4.6
Sheffield	2	2	4	2.2
South Thames	36	15	51	7.6

(Source: **UK Transplant Report 2005**)

Coventry, Bristol or Leicester, you are more likely to be encouraged to have a living donor transplant than if, say, you were living in Plymouth or Sheffield.

It is interesting to not that the number of living donor transplants done in the UK does not seem to have an impact on the overall number of transplants that are performed. So even if the unit down the road from you is doing more living donor transplants, it doesn't mean that you are any more likely to get a transplant (from any source, living or cadaveric). In fact the number of people on the waiting list for a transplant continues to rise at a much faster rate than the rate of increase in the number of transplants performed. This can be seen by the graph on page 140 which shows the number of cadaveric transplants that are performed each year and the number of patients waiting for a transplant each year. More information about this subject can be found on the Transplant UK website (see page 162).

CHOICE – REAL OR NOT?

During the early part of the twenty first century a buzzword has crept into the minds of UK citizens . . . 'choice'. The government wants the people of this country to have a choice of public services: whether that is for transport, schools or hospitals (including Renal Units).

Through the use of the Internet, the press, data collected by organisations such as Ofsted (who report on schools' performance) and the 'star system' in hospitals, it is now relatively easy to find out where better services are available. This system obviously attracts more pupils, customers or patients to the better performing services. The better units will hopefully drive up the standards of the less good, and the public will get the best for themselves and their family.

However, the matter of choice is far more complicated than it might first appear when it comes to the provision of services for the treatment of kidney failure. There are a huge number of factors that affect your choices, some of which are within your control and some, unfortunately which are not.

Availability of resources

As discussed above, there are clearly very different levels of service provided in various parts of the UK. In some areas, you are more likely to be encouraged to have a living donor transplant than in others. Additionally, there are very few renal units in the UK who offer patients home haemodialysis. Although on average, about 75% of dialysis patients are treated with haemodialysis, in some hospitals this is as low as 60% and in others it is as high as 96%. This begs the questions as to whether all kidney patients in the UK actually get a choice of treatment or if treatments are offered depending on the services that are available. If haemodialysis facilities exist in an area, it makes financial sense to have them operating at full capacity.

It is possible for patients to move house so that they live close to a renal unit that is able to offer them their treatment of choice, but this is impractical for most people.

Education and information

If patients are to be offered a true choice of treatment, then that choice should be an informed one. Therefore education and information are vital to the decision making process. In order for patients to receive useful information it should be done in a way that is appropriate for each individual. Some people learn well through reading books and leaflets, others like to use the Internet and some like to watch videos. Many prefer to talk to a healthcare professional or another patient to gain their experience. It's therefore important for the people who are giving the information to be aware of how you like to learn.

People who are diagnosed with kidney failure in good time may spend many years visiting the renal clinic.

Each time they visit, they may see a different doctor. Each doctor could have different levels of experience, which could make their opinions biased against one treatment or another. For example, doctors who have little or no experience of PD (usually because they work within the hospital and PD patients are generally at home, particularly if they are well) may give quite a negative impression of PD.

Time
The amount of time a person has before they start treatment for kidney failure can have a big impact on their 'choice' of treatment. People who are referred to a renal unit months or years before treatment is needed, are far more likely to be given a full programme of education in small frequent sessions. They will be able to go away and think about the information they have been given, ask questions and make informed choices. People who arrive on a renal unit requiring dialysis immediately, however, are much more likely to be offered no choice of treatment and to be started on haemodialysis, usually with temporary access (*see page 70*) which carries a high risk of infection.

It is also true that patients who are referred to the renal unit in plenty of time are much more likely to have a kidney transplant before they actually need dialysis, particularly if they are being treated at a hospital where they actively encourage living donor transplants. However, there are some hospitals that never offer a transplant to a patient before they have started dialysis.

Social circumstances
A person's social situation may also affect their choice of treatment. For example, home dialysis (either PD or haemodialysis) requires some storage space and most people who have home haemodialysis also need some support from a helper.

People who work or do a lot of travelling may choose PD in preference to haemodialysis. However, if you live very close to a renal unit, haemodialysis might be the treatment of choice for you, purely for reasons of convenience.

Making the right choice can be difficult, but it is important to remember that throughout your life with kidney failure, you will probably experience all types of treatment. One may be more appropriate for you at the start of kidney failure. This may change at some stage, say 2–5 years later. The more information you have, the easier it will be to make the right choice at the right time. We hope that this book has given you some information that will help, and the confidence to ask for more.

TRYING TO MAKE IT BETTER
Recent changes in the way health services are organised have been made with the intention of getting rid of the 'postcode lottery' discussed in the previous chapter and making the way healthcare is provided fairer for everybody. Standards for the care everyone with kidney failure should expect from their doctors and nurses have been drawn up. We hope that they will help all patients to receive equally good care – and indeed to complain if they do not receive it.

THE RENAL NATIONAL SERVICE FRAMEWORK
In April 1998 the UK government launched a programme of National Service Frameworks. This was part of a number of measures that were introduced in the NHS Plan to raise quality and decrease variations in service in the NHS. These National Service Frameworks (or NSFs) cover a range of conditions including mental health, cancer and diabetes.

The idea behind the National Service Frameworks is that patients and their doctors should be the ones making choices about health. (All too often, it may

AN EXAMPLE OF A RENAL NETWORK

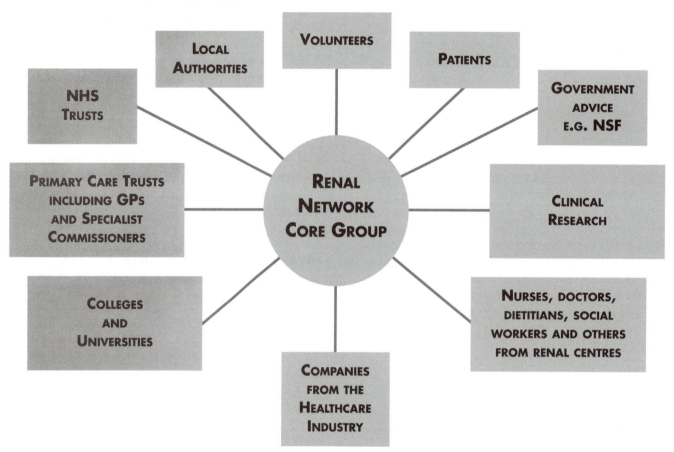

appear that these choices are being made by policy makers). The NSFs also stress the importance of giving local community services and GPs opportunities to improve health in their area.

The Renal National Service Framework (NSF) is in two parts. Part 1 was published in January 2004. It sets out five standards and identifies 30 markers of good practice which the NHS will need to deliver by 2014. These are aimed at helping the health services to manage demand, increase fairness of access – and

improve choice and quality in dialysis and kidney transplant services. Part 2, which was published in 2005, focuses on the prevention of ERF, primary care, and end-of-life care.

The NSF was written and developed by a team of external reference groups (ERGs), which brought together health professionals, patients and carers, health service managers, partner agencies, and other advocates. The Department of Health was also involved in supporting the ERGs and managing the overall process.

The five standards set out in Part 1 are as follows:

Standard 1 – A patient-centred service

'All children, young people and adults with chronic kidney disease are to have access to information that enables them with their carers to make informed decisions and encourages partnership in decision making, with an agreed care plan that supports them in managing their condition to achieve the best possible quality of life.'

Standard 2 – Preparation and Choice

'All children, young people and adults approaching established renal failure are to receive timely preparation for renal replacement therapy so the complications and progression of their disease are minimised, and their choice of clinically appropriate treatment options is maximised.'

Standard 3 – Elective dialysis access surgery

'All children, young people and adults with established renal failure are to have timely and appropriate surgery for permanent vascular or peritoneal dialysis access, which is monitored and maintained to achieve its maximum longevity.'

Standard 4 – Dialysis

'Renal services are to ensure the delivery of high quality clinically appropriate forms of dialysis which are designed around individual needs and preferences and are available to patients of all ages throughout their lives.'

Standard 5 – Transplantation

'All children, young people and adults likely to benefit from a kidney transplant are to receive a high quality service which supports them in managing their transplant and enables them to achieve the best possible quality of life.'

Part 2 focuses on 'Quality requirements', as listed below:

Quality requirement 1: Prevention and early detection of chronic kidney disease

This quality requirement stresses the importance of identifying kidney failure early, especially where people are at a higher than average risk of developing kidney disease of having it undiagnosed. Early detection will give doctors the best possible chance of helping the person to manage his or her health in such a way that their kidney function will be preserved for as long as possible.

Quality requirement 2: Minimising the progression and consequences of chronic kidney disease

This stresses the importance of following up and monitoring the health of people with chronic kidney disease in order to reduce the risk of progression and complications.

Quality requirement 3: Acute renal failure

People at risk of, or suffering from, acute renal failure need to be identified promptly, with hospital services delivering high quality, clinically appropriate care in partnership with specialised renal teams.

Quality requirement 4: End of life care

People with established renal failure must be treated with honesty and respect and given appropriate information about the choices available to them. Plans for care in the period towards the end of life should be agreed by health professionals in consultation with the individuals themselves, so that any palliative care plan is built specifically around their own needs and preferences.

The NSF goes on to make the point that these standards and quality requirements apply to *all* people with, or at risk of, kidney failure. In some cases, for example, children and young people and some older people, they will also apply (in varying degrees) to families, guardians or carers.

DELIVERING RENAL SERVICES

Traditionally services for people with ERF have been centred around hospital haemodialysis in a limited number of main renal units where renal consultants, inpatient and investigative facilities are based. In the 1970s and 1980s programmes of home haemodialysis and peritoneal dialysis were established. The 1990s saw the development of a 'hub and spoke' model with many main renal units supported by one or more satellite haemodialysis units closer to patients' homes. In some cases the traditional hub and spoke model has evolved into a so-called 'clinical network', whereby the majority of renal care is as close to patients' homes as possible.

The renal NSF aims to help renal services to build on the most successful elements of these models, while providing a more responsive service closer to home. More about the NSF for renal patients and what it might mean for you can be found on the Department of Health's website (see *page 160* for address details).

THE PATIENTS' ROLE IN ALL THIS

The Expert Patient Programme

The Expert Patient Programme is an NHS based patient-training programme that was set up in 2002. It is designed to help people to cope with long-term illnesses better by teaching them to look after themselves. To become an Expert Patient you need to attend a "Self-Management" course that will help you to:

- Manage your medication
- Reduce levels of depression, fatigue and anxiety

- Improve communication with healthcare professionals such as specialist doctors and nurses
- Improve relaxation, exercise and diet
- Help you to be independent and more mobile
- Improve your job or voluntary work prospects
- Improve or maintain your quality of life

The course takes place over 6 weeks with one 2-hour session each week. So far the Expert Patient Programme has shown the following benefits:

- Fewer consultations
- Shorter waiting lists
- Fewer missed appointments
- Prescription cost savings
- Better communication with patients and healthcare providers
- Fewer admissions to hospital

To find out about The Expert Patient Programme in your area, visit www.expertpatients.nhs.uk

Patients' voices, patients' rights

With the publication of the Renal NSF comes a great opportunity for patients and relatives or carers to become involved in improving the provision of renal services. Where NSF standards are not being met (and there is a shortfall in available treatment), or where patients feel they are not getting the choices they deserve, there are some things they can do about it. If you, or someone you care about, is in this position here are some suggestions:

- Become involved in your local renal network
- If you feel that local services are not up to

standard, why not write to your local newspaper? Publicity is a powerful tool.

- Join your local Kidney Patients' Association if there is one. If there is not one, consider whether you might be the person to start one.

- It is also a good idea to join the National Kidney Federation (NKF) which speaks for all kidney patients and has links with the All-Party Parliamentary Group for Kidneys (APPGK) – a group of MPs who fight for resources for kidney patients.

- Write to your MP or, even better; visit his or her local surgery. Not all politicians are aware of the major problems in British kidney medicine.

Whether you do one or all of these, keep at it!

KEY FACTS

1 There is simply not enough care for patients with kidney disease throughout the UK. A major reason for this is inadequate funding which makes providing and staffing a renal unit very difficult.

2 The amount and type of dialysis provided around the country varies significantly.

3 There is also a shortage of kidneys for transplant. More kidneys from living donors are needed; and relatives, partners and friends should be actively encouraged to consider donating a kidney to a loved one.

3 There is more information out there now, allowing patients to make choices, with regards to their care. It is debatable whether the choices are real.

5 A National Service Framework (NSF) for the care of renal patients has been developed. The aim of this is to give responsibility for care back to patients and their doctors.

6 Part 1 gives 5 standards and 30 markers of good practice to ensure that services for dialysis and transplant patients are of an appropriate standard everywhere in the UK.

7 Part 2 of the renal NSF focuses on the prevention of established renal failure, primary care, and care at the end of life. It lists four quality requirements relevant to these areas.

8 The Expert Patient Programme enables patients to help themselves and each other.

9 Patients have a right to be heard. Joining relevant organisations and writing to the local paper or your MP is a good place to start.

GLOSSARY

This glossary provides brief explanations of the various technical words and abbreviations used in this book. Words printed in *italic* type have their own glossary entry.

Abdomen The lower part of the trunk, below the chest. Commonly called the tummy or belly.

Access A method of gaining entry to the bloodstream to allow *dialysis*. Access methods used for *haemodialysis* include a *catheter*, *fistula* or *graft*.

Acid A chemical that builds up in the blood in *kidney failure*.

Acute A word meaning short term and of rapid onset, usually requiring a rapid response.

Adequacy This term is used to describe the tests that are used to see how much *dialysis* a patient is getting. Samples of the *dialysis fluid*, blood and samples of *urine* are used to measure the dialysis adequacy.

Albumin A type of *protein* that occurs in the blood. Low blood levels may be linked to *malnutrition*.

Alfacalcidol A *vitamin D* supplement.

ALG Abbreviation for anti-lymphocyte globulin, a strong treatment against the *rejection* of a *transplant kidney*.

Alkali A substance that is the chemical opposite of an acid.

Alpha-blocker A type of *blood pressure* tablet – examples include doxazosin and terazosin.

Aluminium hydroxide A commonly-used type of *phosphate binder*, used to help prevent and treat *renal bone disease*. An example of aluminium hydroxide is Alu-Cap.

Amino acids Substances from which *proteins* are built up.

Anaemia A shortage of *red blood cells* in the body, causing tiredness, shortness of breath and pale skin. One of the functions of the *kidneys* is to make *erythropoietin*, which stimulates the *bone marrow* to make *blood cells*. In *kidney failure*, EPO is not made, and anaemia results.

Angiogram A type of X-ray that uses a special dye to show the *blood vessels*. The dye is put into the blood vessels via a tube that is inserted into the groin and passed up to the *kidneys*.

Angiotensin II (A2) antagonist A type of blood pressure tablet that can make can make kidney function worse, although it can be useful in certain situations. Also known as an ARB.

Angiotensin-converting enzyme (ACE) inhibitor A type of *blood pressure* tablet that can make kidney function worse, although it is useful in certain situations.

Ankle oedema An abnormal build-up of fluid in the skin around the ankles. It is an early sign of *fluid overload*.

Antibiotic drugs A group of drugs used to treat infections caused by *bacteria*.

Antibodies Substances that normally help the body to fight infection. They are made by *white blood cells*. After a *transplant*, antibodies can attack the new *kidney* and cause *rejection*.

Antigen A type of *protein* that occurs on the outer surface of all the cells in a person's body. Antigens act as a 'friendly face' for the cells. The *immune system* normally recognises the friendly face of the body's own *cells*, and does not attack or reject them.

APD Abbreviation for automated peritoneal dialysis. A form of *peritoneal dialysis* that uses a machine to drain the *dialysis fluid* out of the patient and replace it with fresh solution. APD is usually carried out overnight while the patient sleeps.

Arteries *Blood vessels* that carry blood from the heart to the rest of the body.

Artificial kidney Another name for the *dialyser* or filtering unit of a *dialysis machine*.

ATG Abbreviation for anti-thymocyte globulin, a strong treatment against the *rejection* of a *transplant kidney*.

Atheroma Deposits of *cholesterol* and other fats that cause furring and narrowing of the *arteries* (also called atherosclerosis).

Azathioprine An *immuno-suppressant drug* used to prevent the rejection of a *transplant kidney*.

Bacteria A type of germ. Bacteria are microscopically tiny, single-celled organisms capable of independent life. Most are harmless, but some cause disease.

Beta-blockers Tablets that slow down the heart rate and lower blood pressure. Examples are atenolol, bisoprolol, metoprolol and propranolol.

Bicarbonate A substance that is normally present in the blood which is measured in the *biochemistry blood test*. A low blood level of bicarbonate shows there is too much *acid* in the blood.

Biochemistry blood test A test that measures the blood levels of various different substances. Substances measured in people with *kidney failure* usually include *sodium*, *potassium*, *glucose*, *urea*, *creatinine*, *bicarbonate*, *calcium*, *phosphate* and *albumin*.

Biopsy A test involving the removal of a small piece of an organ or other body *tissue* and its examination under a microscope. A *kidney biopsy* is sometimes used to try and establish the cause of *kidney failure*. Biopsies are also used to check whether a transplanted *kidney* is being rejected.

BK virus A recently-discovered virus that can cause a transplanted kidney to work less well, or affect the blood.

Bladder The organ in which *urine* is stored before being passed from the body.

Blood cells The microscopically tiny units that form the solid part of the blood. There are three main types: *red blood cells*, *white blood cells* and *platelets*.

Blood group An inherited characteristic of *red blood cells*. The common classification is based on whether or not a person has certain *antigens* (called A and B) on their cells. People belong to one of four blood groups, called A, B, AB and O.

Blood level A measurement of the amount of a particular substance in the blood, sometimes expressed in mmol/l (millimoles per litre) or μmol/l (micromoles per litre) of blood.

Blood pressure The pressure that the blood exerts against the walls of the *arteries* as it flows through them. Blood pressure measurements consist of two numbers. The first shows the *systolic blood pressure*, the second, the *diastolic blood pressure*. Normal blood pressure is 130/80 or less for most people. One of the functions of the *kidneys* is to help control the blood pressure. In *kidney failure*, the blood pressure tends to be high.

Blood vessels The tubes that carry blood around the body. The main blood vessels are the *arteries* and *veins*.

Bone marrow The 'runny' part in the middle of some bones, where blood *cells* are made.

BP Abbreviation for *blood pressure*.

Brain death A term indicating that the entire brain has permanently stopped working, and that further life is possible only on a life support machine. A person must be diagnosed brain dead before their organs can be removed for a *cadaveric transplant*.

Cadaveric transplant A *transplant kidney* removed from someone who has died.

Calcium A mineral that strengthens the bones. It is contained in some foods, including dairy products. It is stored in the bones and is present in the blood. The *kidneys* normally help to keep calcium in the bones. In *kidney failure*, calcium drains out of the bones, and the level of calcium in the blood also falls.

Calcium acetate An alternative to calcium carbonate.

Calcium antagonist A type of blood pressure tablet that can cause 'ankle swelling'. Examples include amlodipine and nifedipine.

Calcium carbonate A commonly used type of *phosphate binder*, used to help prevent and treat *renal bone disease*. An example of calcium carbonate is Calcichew.

Candida albicans A fungus that sometimes causes *peritonitis* in patients on *peritoneal dialysis*.

CAPD Abbreviation for continuous ambulatory peritoneal dialysis.

A continuous form of *peritoneal dialysis* in which patients perform the exchanges of *dialysis fluid* by hand. The fluid is usually exchanged four times during the day, and is left inside the patient overnight.

Catheter A flexible plastic tube used to enter the interior of the body. A catheter is one of the access options for patients on *haemodialysis*. For patients on *peritoneal dialysis*, a catheter allows *dialysis fluid* to be put into and removed from the *peritoneal cavity*. A catheter may also be used to drain *urine* from the *bladder*.

Cells The tiny units from which all living things are built up. Most cells have some common features (including a nucleus that is the cell's control centre, and an outer membrane or skin that gives the cell its shape). Cells in different parts of the body look different from each other and perform different functions (for example, skin cells are very different from blood cells).

Cholesterol A *lipid* (fat) that is a major contributor to *atheroma*.

Chronic A word meaning long term and of slow onset, not usually requiring immediate action.

Ciclosporin An *immuno-suppressant drug* used to prevent the *rejection* of a *transplant kidney*.

Clearance The removal of the toxic waste products of food from the body. Clearance is one of the two main functions of the *kidneys*. In *kidney failure*, clearance is inadequate, and *toxins* from food build up in the blood.

CMV Abbreviation for *cytomegalovirus*.

Creatinine A waste substance produced by the muscles when they are used. The higher the blood creatinine level, the worse the *kidneys* (or *dialysis* or kidney *transplant*) are working.

Creatinine clearance test A test that measures how effectively the kidneys are working. It involves comparing the creatinine level in the blood to that in the urine. It is normally around 100 mls/min, which approximates to 100 % of normal kidney function. It is similar to the eGFR and is used mainly in the pre-dialysis period.

Cross-match The final blood test before a *transplant operation* is performed. It checks whether the patient has any *antibodies* to the donor *kidney*. The operation can proceed only if the cross-match is negative (i.e. no antibodies are found).

CT scan Abbreviation for a computed tomography scan. An investigation that uses a computer to build up a picture from a series of low-intensity X-rays.

Cytomegalovirus (CMV) A *virus* that normally causes only a mild 'flu-like illness. In people with a *kidney transplant* (and in other people whose *immune system* is suppressed), CMV can cause a more serious illness, affecting the lungs, liver and blood.

Dehydration A condition in which the body does not contain enough water to function properly. Dehydration often occurs with low *blood pressure*, which causes weakness and dizziness.

Diabetes mellitus A condition (also known as 'sugar diabetes' or simply as diabetes) in which there is too much

sugar in the blood. Whether this type of diabetes is controlled by insulin, tablets or diet, it can cause *kidney failure*. This happens most often to people who have had diabetes for longer than 10 years.

Diabetic nephropathy Kidney failure caused by *diabetes mellitus*.

Dialyser The filtering unit of a *dialysis machine*. It provides the *dialysis membrane* for patients on *haemodialysis*. The dialyser removes body wastes and excess water from the blood in a similar way to a normal *kidney*.

Dialysis An artificial process by which the toxic waste products of food and excess water are removed from the body. Dialysis therefore takes over some of the work normally performed by healthy *kidneys*. The name dialysis comes from a Greek word meaning 'to separate' – i.e. to separate out the 'bad things' in the blood from the 'good things'.

Dialysis fluid The liquid that provides the 'container' into which toxic waste products and excess water pass during *dialysis* for removal from the body.

Dialysis machine The machine used to perform *haemodialysis*. It includes a *dialyser*, which filters the patient's blood. The machine helps to pump the patient's blood through the dialyser, and monitors the dialysis process as it takes place.

Dialysis membrane A thin layer of tissue or plastic with many tiny holes in it, through which the process of *dialysis* takes place. In *peritoneal dialysis*, the patient's *peritoneum* provides the dialysis membrane. For *haemodialysis*, the dialysis membrane is made of plastic. In each case, the membrane keeps the *dialysis fluid* separate from the blood (essential because dialysis fluid is toxic if it flows directly into the blood). However, the tiny holes in the membrane make it *semi-permeable*, allowing water and various substances to pass through it.

Diastolic blood pressure A *blood pressure* reading taken when the heart is relaxed. It is taken after the *systolic blood pressure*, and is the second figure in a blood pressure measurement. It should be 80 mmHg or less.

Diffusion A process by which substances pass from a stronger to a weaker solution. Diffusion is one of the key processes in *dialysis* (the other is *ultrafiltration*). During dialysis, body wastes such as *creatinine* pass from the blood into the *dialysis fluid*. At the same time, useful substances such as *bicarbonate* and *calcium* pass from the dialysis fluid into the blood.

Diuretic drugs The medical name for water tablets. These drugs increase the amount of *urine* that is passed. Two commonly used diuretics are *furosemide* and bumetanide.

Donor A person who donates (gives) an organ to another person (the recipient).

Donor kidney A *kidney* that has been donated.

Doppler scan A type of *ultrasound scan* (sound-wave picture) that provides information about blood flow through the *arteries*.

ECG Abbreviation for *electrocardiogram*.

ECHO Abbreviation for *echocardiogram*.

Echocardiogram (ECHO) A type of *ultrasound scan* (sound-wave picture) that shows how well the heart is working.

eGFR Estimated *glomerular filtration rate*. The term is generally applied to a test which measures how well the kidneys are working. It is normally around 100 mls/min, which approximates to 100 % of normal kidney function. It is similar to the creatinine clearance test and is used mainly in the pre-dialysis period.

Electrocardiogram (ECG) A test that shows the electrical activity within the heart.

End-stage renal failure (ESRF) An alternative name for *established renal failure*.

End-stage renal disease (ESRD) An alternative name for *established renal failure*.

EPO Abbreviation for *erythropoietin*.

ERF Abbreviation for *established renal failure*.

Erythropoietin (EPO) A *hormone*, made by the *kidneys*, which stimulates the *bone marrow* to produce red blood cells.

Established renal failure (ERF) A term for advanced chronic *kidney failure*. People who develop ERF will die within a *few weeks* unless treated by *dialysis* or *transplantation*. These treatments control ERF but cannot cure it. Once a patient has developed ERF, they will always have it, even after a *transplant*.

ESRF Abbreviation for *end-stage renal failure*.

ESRD Abbreviation for *end-stage renal disease*.

Exit site The point where a *catheter* comes out through the skin. Exit site infections can be a problem for *peritoneal dialysis* patients.

Ferritin A substance in the blood that indicates how much *iron* is present. The more iron there is in the body, the higher the level of ferritin in the blood.

Fistula An enlarged *vein*, usually at the wrist or elbow, that gives access to the bloodstream for *haemodialysis*. The fistula is created by a surgeon in a small operation. It is done by joining a vein to an *artery*. This increases the flow of blood through the vein and causes it to enlarge, making it suitable for haemodialysis needles.

FK506 Another name for *tacrolimus*.

Flucloxacillin An antibiotic used to treat *exit site* infections of *peritoneal dialysis* and *haemodialysis* catheters.

Fluid overload A condition in which the body contains too much water. It is caused by drinking too much fluid, or not losing enough. Fluid overload occurs in *kidney failure* because one of the main functions of the *kidneys* is to remove excess water. Fluid overload often occurs with high *blood pressure*. Excess fluid first gathers around the ankles (*ankle oedema*) and may later settle in the lungs (*pulmonary oedema*).

Furosemide A commonly used *diuretic*.

Gentamicin An antibiotic used to treat *peritonitis*.

GFR An abbreviation for glomerular filtration rate, also the name of a test which indicates how effectively the kidneys get rid of waste by measuring the number of millilitres of blood the kidneys are able to filter in one minute.

Glomerulonephritis Inflammation of the glomeruli, which is one of the causes of *kidney failure*.

Glomerulus One of the tiny filtering units inside the *kidney*.

Glucose A type of sugar. There is normally a small amount of glucose in the blood. This amount is not usually increased in people with *kidney failure* unless they also have *diabetes mellitus*. Glucose is the main substance in *peritoneal dialysis* fluid, drawing excess water into the *dialysis fluid* from the blood by *osmosis*.

Graft A type of access for *haemodialysis*. The graft is a small plastic tube that connects an *artery* to a *vein*. It is inserted into the arm or leg by a surgeon. *Haemodialysis* needles are inserted into the graft, which can be used many hundreds of times.

Haemodialysis A form of *dialysis* in which the blood is cleaned outside the body, in a machine called a *dialysis machine* or *kidney machine*. The machine contains a filter called the dialyser or artificial kidney. Each dialysis session lasts for 3–5 hours, and sessions are usually needed 2–3 times a week.

Haemodialysis catheter A plastic tube used to gain access to the bloodstream for *haemodialysis*.

Haemodialysis unit The part of a hospital where patients go for *haemodialysis*.

Haemoglobin (Hb) A substance in red blood cells that carries oxygen around the body. Blood levels of haemoglobin are measured to look for *anaemia*. A low Hb level indicates anaemia.

Hb Abbreviation for *haemoglobin*.

Heart-beating donor A term used to describe a donor whose heart is still beating after *brain death* has occurred. Most, but not all, *cadaveric transplants* come from heart-beating donors.

Hepatitis An infection of the liver, usually caused by a *virus*. Two main types, called hepatitis B and hepatitis C, can be passed on by blood contact. This means that *dialysis* patients, especially those on *haemodialysis*, have an increased risk of getting these infections. Care is taken to reduce this risk, and regular virus checks are made on all kidney patients.

HIV Human immunodeficiency virus, the virus that causes AIDS. Tests for this virus are carried out before a patient can have a *transplant*. This is because HIV may be present and inactive in the patient's body but can be activated by the transplant and *immuno-suppressant drugs*, and cause illness.

Home haemodialysis Treatment on a *dialysis machine* installed in a patient's own home. For home haemodialysis to be considered, the patient must have a partner or friend who is able to supervise *every* dialysis session.

Hormones Substances that act as chemical messengers in the body. They are produced in parts of the body called endocrine glands. Hormones travel around the body in the blood, and control how other parts of the body work. For example, *parathyroid hormone* from the *parathyroid glands* in the neck affects *kidney* function.

Hyperparathyroidism A disorder in which the *parathyroid glands* make too much *parathyroid hormone*.

Immune system The body's natural defence system. It includes organs (such as the spleen and appendix), lymph nodes (including the 'glands' in the neck) and specialist *white blood cells* called *lymphocytes*. The immune system protects the body from infections, foreign bodies and cancer. To prevent *rejection* of a *transplant kidney*, it is necessary for patients to take *immuno-suppressant drugs*.

Immuno-suppressant drugs A group of drugs used to dampen down the *immune system* to prevent *rejection* of a *transplant kidney*. Commonly used examples are *ciclosporin, azathioprine, prednisolone, tacrolimus* and *mycophenolate mofetil*.

Intravenous pyelogram (IVP) A special X-ray of the *kidneys*.
A dye that shows up on X-rays is used to show the drainage system of the kidneys. The dye is injected into the patient's arm, travels in the blood to the kidneys, and is passed from the body in the *urine*.

Iron A substance that is necessary to prevent *anaemia*. A low blood *ferritin* indicates low levels of iron in the body.

IVP Abbreviation for *intravenous pyelogram*.

Kidneys The two bean-shaped body organs where *urine* is made. They are located at the back of the body, below the ribs. The two main functions of the kidneys are to remove toxic wastes and to remove *excess water* from the body. The kidneys also help to control *blood pressure*, help to control the manufacture of *red blood cells*, and help to keep the bones strong and healthy.

Kidney biopsy Removal of a small piece of *kidney* through a hollow needle for examination under a microscope. It is needed to diagnose some causes of kidney failure, including *nephritis*. It is also used to check whether a transplanted kidney is being rejected.

Kidney donor A person who gives a *kidney* for *transplantation*.

Kidney failure A condition in which the *kidneys* are less able than normal to perform their functions of removing toxic wastes, removing excess water, helping to control *blood pressure*, helping to control *red blood cell* manufacture and helping to keep the bones strong and healthy. Kidney failure can be *acute* or *chronic*. Advanced chronic kidney failure is called *established renal failure* or *ERF*.

Kidney machine Another name for a *dialysis machine*.

Kidney transplant An alternative name for a *transplant kidney*, or for the *transplant operation* during which a new *kidney* is given to the recipient.

LFTs Abbreviation for *liver function tests*.

Line infection A term for an infection of a *haemodialysis catheter* (or line).

Lipids Another name for fats. People with *kidney failure* tend to have raised lipid levels in the blood.

Liver function tests (LFTs) Blood tests that show how well the liver is working. They often appear at the bottom of the *biochemistry blood test* results. Some people with *kidney failure* also have liver problems.

Living related transplant (LRT) A *transplant kidney* donated (given) by a living relative of the recipient. A well-matched living related transplant is likely to last longer than either a *living unrelated transplant* or a *cadaveric transplant*.

Living unrelated transplant (LURT) A *kidney transplant* from a living person who is biologically unrelated to the recipient (such as a husband or wife).

LRT Abbreviation for a *living related transplant*.

LURT Abbreviation for a *living unrelated transplant*.

Lymphocytes Specialist *white blood cells* that form part of the *immune system*.

Malnutrition Loss of body weight, usually due to not eating enough (especially foods providing *protein* and energy). Malnutrition is the major nutritional problem of *dialysis* patients.

Marker A substance that is known to occur in the presence of another substance. Both *creatinine* and *urea* are markers for many less easily measurable substances in the blood. The higher the blood levels of these marker substances, the higher also are the levels of harmful *toxins* in the blood.

Membrane A thin, skin-like layer, resembling a piece of 'cling film'. The *peritoneum* is a natural membrane used as the *dialysis membrane* in *peritoneal dialysis*. In *haemodialysis*, the dialysis membrane is a plastic membrane inside the *dialyser*.

Methylprednisolone A strong version of *prednisolone*, a drug used to prevent or treat the *rejection* of a *transplant kidney*.

mmol/l Abbreviation for millimoles per litre. A unit used to measure the blood levels of many substances. *Creatinine* is measured in smaller units called micromoles per litre (µmol/l).

Molecule The smallest unit that a substance can be divided into without causing a change in the chemical nature of the substance.

MRI scan Abbreviation for magnetic resonance imaging scan, a scanning technique that uses magnetism, radiowaves and a computer to produce high-quality pictures of the body's interior.

Mycophenolate mofetil A new *immuno-suppressant drug*. Sometimes used as an alternative to *azathioprine*.

Nephr- Prefix meaning relating to the *kidneys*.

Nephrectomy An operation to remove a *kidney* from the body. A bilateral nephrectomy is an operation to remove both kidneys.

Nephritis A general term for inflammation of the *kidneys*. Also used as an abbreviation for *glomerulonephritis*. A *kidney biopsy* is needed to diagnose nephritis.

Nephrologist Another name for a kidney doctor.

Nephrology The study of the *kidneys*.

NICE Abbreviation for National Institute for Health and Clinical Excellence, and the name by which this body is commonly known. NICE looks at whether new treatments are effective and issues guidelines for good practice.

Non-heart-beating donor A donor whose heart is not beating after death, for example after having had a heart attack in casualty when resuscitation has failed. A few cadaveric *kidneys* come from this source.

Nuclear medicine scan Another name for a *radio-isotope scan*. Examples include DMSA, DTPA, and MAG-3 scans.

Obstructive nephropathy Blockage to the drainage system of the *kidney*, through which the *urine* passes.

Oedema An abnormal build-up of fluid, mainly water, in the body. People with *kidney failure* are prone to *fluid overload*, leading to oedema. The two most common places for water to collect in the body are around the ankles (*ankle oedema*) and in the lungs (*pulmonary oedema*).

OKT3 Abbreviation for orthoclone K T-cell receptor 3 antibody, a strong treatment for the *rejection* of a *transplant*.

Organ A part of the body that consists of different types of *tissue*, and that performs a particular function. Examples include the *kidneys*, heart and brain.

Osmosis The process by which water moves from a weaker to a stronger solution through tiny holes in a *semi-permeable* membrane. In *peritoneal dialysis*, it is osmosis that causes excess water to pass from the blood into the *dialysis fluid*.

Parathyroidectomy An operation to remove the *parathyroid glands*.

Parathyroid glands Four pea-sized glands near the thyroid gland at the front of the neck. They produce *parathyroid hormone*.

Parathyroid hormone (PTH) A hormone produced by the *parathyroid glands*, which helps control blood levels of *calcium*. When the level of calcium in the blood is low, PTH boosts it by causing calcium to drain from the bones into the blood. PTH is the best long-term indicator of the severity of *renal bone disease*.

PCKD Abbreviation for *polycystic kidney disease*.

PD Abbreviation for *peritoneal dialysis*.

PD catheter A plastic tube through which *dialysis fluid* for *peritoneal dialysis* is put into, and removed from, the *peritoneal cavity*. The catheter is about 30 centimetres (12 inches) long, and as wide as a pencil. A small operation is needed to insert the catheter permanently into the *abdomen*.

Peritoneal cavity The area between the two layers of the *peritoneum* inside the *abdomen*. The peritoneal cavity contains the abdominal organs, including the stomach, liver and bowels. It normally contains only about 100 ml of liquid, but expands easily to provide a reservoir for the *dialysis fluid* in *peritoneal dialysis*.

Peritoneal dialysis (PD) A form of *dialysis* that takes place inside the patient's *peritoneal cavity*, using the *peritoneum* as the *dialysis membrane*. Bags of *dialysis fluid*, containing *glucose* (sugar) and various other substances, are drained in and out of the peritoneal cavity via a PD catheter.

Peritoneal equilibration test (PET) A measurement of the rate at which *toxins* pass out of the blood into the dialysis fluid during *peritoneal dialysis* (PD). Patients are described as 'high transporters' (if the toxins move quickly) and 'low transporters' (if the toxins move more slowly). The test is used to assess a patient's suitability for different types of PD.

Peritoneum A natural membrane that lines the inside of the wall of the *abdomen* and that covers all the abdominal organs (the stomach, bowels, liver, etc.). The peritoneum provides the *dialysis membrane* for *peritoneal dialysis*. It has a large surface area, contains many tiny holes and has a good blood supply.

Peritonitis Inflammation of the *peritoneum*, caused by an infection. People on *peritoneal dialysis* risk getting peritonitis if they touch the connection between their *peritoneal dialysis* catheter and the bags of *dialysis fluid*. Most attacks are easily treated with *antibiotic drugs*.

PET In this context, an abbreviation for the *peritoneal equilibration test*. (The abbreviation PET in PET scan is short for positron emission tomography.)

Phosphate A mineral that helps *calcium* to strengthen the bones. Phosphate is obtained from foods such as dairy products, nuts and meat. The *kidneys* normally help to keep the right amount of phosphate in the blood. In *kidney failure*, phosphate tends to build up in the blood. High phosphate levels occur with low calcium levels in people with *renal bone disease*.

Phosphate binders Tablets that help prevent a build-up of *phosphate* in the body. Phosphate binders combine with phosphate in food so that it passes it out of the body in the faeces. The most commonly used phosphate binders are *calcium carbonate* and *aluminium hydroxide*.

Plasma The liquid part of the blood in which the blood *cells* float.

Platelets A type of blood *cell* that helps the blood to clot.

Polycystic kidney disease (PCKD) An inherited disease (a disease that runs in families) in which both kidneys are full ('poly' means 'many') of cysts (abnormal fluid-filled lumps). PCKD is one of the causes of *kidney failure*. It is diagnosed by an *ultrasound scan*.

Potassium A mineral that is normally present in the blood, and which is measured in the *biochemistry blood test*. Either too much or too little potassium can be dangerous, causing the heart to stop. People with *kidney failure* may need to restrict the amount of potassium in their diet.

Prednisolone A drug used to prevent or treat the *rejection* of a *transplant kidney*.

Proteins Chemical components of the body, formed from *amino acids*. The body needs supplies of protein in the diet to build muscles and to repair itself.

PTH Abbreviation for *parathyroid hormone*.

Pulmonary oedema A serious condition in which fluid builds up in the lungs, causing breathlessness. People with *kidney failure* develop pulmonary oedema if *fluid overload* is not treated promptly.

Pyelonephritis Inflammation of the drainage system of the *kidneys*, one of the causes of *kidney failure*. It can be diagnosed by an ultrasound scan, an intravenous pyelogram or a nuclear medicine scan.

Radio-isotope scan A method of obtaining pictures of the body's interior, also called a *radio-nuclide scan* or *nuclear medicine scan*. A small amount of a mildly radioactive substance is either swallowed or injected into the bloodstream. The substance gathers in certain parts of the body, which then show up on pictures taken by a special machine.

Radio-nuclide scan Another name for a *radio-isotope scan*.

Recipient In the context of *transplantation*, a person who receives an organ from another person (the donor).

Red blood cells *Cells* in the blood which carry oxygen from the lungs around the body.

Reflux The movement of a liquid, such as *urine*, in the opposite direction to normal. The word 'reflux' is sometimes used to mean *reflux nephropathy*.

Reflux nephropathy A condition in which *urine* passes back up from the *bladder*, through the *ureters*, to the *kidneys*, where it can cause infections. It occurs because a valve that normally prevents the backflow of urine from the bladder is faulty. Reflux nephropathy is one of the causes of *kidney failure*.

Rejection The process by which a patient's *immune system* recognises a *transplant kidney* (or other transplanted organ) as not its 'own', and then tries to destroy it and remove it from the body. Rejection can be *acute* or *chronic*.

Renal Adjective meaning relating to the *kidneys*.

Renal bone disease A complication of *kidney failure*, in which bone health is affected by abnormally low blood levels of *calcium* and *vitamin D*, and high levels of *phosphate*. Without treatment, renal bone disease can result in bone pain and fractures.

Renal unit A hospital department that treats disorders of the *kidneys*.

Renovascular disease Atheroma affecting the *blood vessels* that supply the kidneys ('reno' means relating to the kidney, and 'vascular' means relating to the blood vessels). Renovascular disease is a common cause of *kidney failure* in older patients.

Residual renal function (RRF) The amount of kidney function that a patient on dialysis has. This varies from patient to patient. It is likely the RRF will reduce over a period of time, and in many patients, it eventually disappears altogether. A *creatinine clearance test* is used to assess RRF.

Rifampicin An *antibiotic drug* used to treat long-term *exit site* infections of *peritoneal dialysis* catheters.

Rigors Cold shivers that sometimes occur with a fever. They can be a symptom of an infected *haemodialysis catheter*.

RRF Abbreviation for *residual renal function*.

Satellite haemodialysis unit A place where some patients go for *haemodialysis* away from the main hospital *renal unit*. Satellite units have relatively few nurses, and are suitable only for healthy patients, who do some of the haemodialysis preparation themselves. These units tend to be more easily accessible to patients than most main hospital buildings.

Scan One of several techniques for obtaining pictures of the body's interior without using conventional X-rays. Examples include *CT scans*, *MRI scans*, *radio-isotope scans* and *ultrasound scans*.

Semi-permeable An adjective, often used to describe a *membrane*, meaning that it will allow some but not all substances to pass through it. Substances with smaller *molecules* will pass through the holes in the membrane, whereas substances with larger molecules will not.

Sirolimus A new immunosuppressant drug which is an alternative to ciclosporin or tacrolimus.

Sodium A mineral that is normally present in the blood, and which is measured in the *biochemistry blood test*. Sodium levels are not usually a problem for people with *kidney failure* and are quite easily controlled by *dialysis*.

Sphygmomanometer The instrument used to measure *blood pressure*.

Staphylococcus One of a group of *bacteria* responsible for various infections (often called 'staph' infections). A common cause of *peritonitis* in patients on *peritoneal dialysis*, and of *line infections* in *haemodialysis* patients.

Statins A group of drugs that reduce lipid levels in the blood, especially cholesterol. Examples include atorvastatin and simvastatin.

Systolic blood pressure A *blood pressure* reading taken when the heart squeezes as it beats. The systolic blood pressure is measured before the *diastolic blood pressure* and is the first figure in a blood pressure measurement.

Tacrolimus An *immuno-suppressant drug*, also known as FK506, which is an alternative to *ciclosporin*.

Tissue A collection of similar *cells* that share a similar function, such as skin cells or *kidney cells*.

Tissue type A set of inherited characteristics on the surface of *cells*. Each person's tissue type has six components (three from each parent). Although there are only three main sorts of tissue type characteristic (called A, B and DR), each of these comes in 20 or more different versions. Given the large number of possibilities, it is unusual for there to be an exact tissue type match between a *transplant kidney* and its recipient. However, the more characteristics that match, the more likely a *transplant* is to succeed.

Tissue typing A blood test that identifies a person's *tissue type*.

Toxins Poisons. One of the main functions of the *kidneys* is to remove toxins from the blood (a process known as *clearance*).

Transplant A term used to mean either a *transplant kidney* (or other transplant organ) or a *transplant operation*.

Transplantation The replacement of an organ in the body by another person's organ. Many different organs can now be successfully transplanted, including the *kidneys*, liver, bowel, heart, lungs, pancreas, skin and bones.

Transplant kidney A *kidney* removed from one person (the donor) and given to another person (the recipient). Transplant kidneys may be either *cadaveric transplants*, *living related transplants* or *living unrelated transplants*.

Transplant operation The surgical operation by which a patient is given a donated organ. The operation to insert a *transplant kidney* takes about 2–3 hours. The new *kidney* is placed lower in the *abdomen* than the patient's own kidneys, which are usually left in place. *Blood vessels* attached to the transplant kidney are connected to the patient's blood supply, and the new kidney's *ureter* is connected to the patient's *bladder*.

Transplant waiting list A system that seeks to find the 'right' transplant organ for the 'right' patient. It is co-ordinated nationally by *UKT*, whose computer compares patients' details (including *blood group* and *tissue type*) with those of cadaveric organs that become available. The average waiting time for a *cadaveric transplant kidney* is about 2 years.

Tuberculosis A bacterium that can cause long-term infections. It is an unusual source of PD peritonitis.

Tunnel infection A possible problem for patients on *peritoneal dialysis* (PD). It occurs when an infection spreads from the *exit site* into the 'tunnel' (i.e. the route of the PD catheter through the abdominal wall).

UKT Abbreviation for United Kingdom Transplant, based in Bristol. This is the national co-ordinator for *cadaveric transplants* in the UK.

ULTRA Abbreviation for Unrelated Living Transplant Regulatory Authority. This government body must give approval to all *living unrelated transplants*.

Ultrafiltration The removal of excess water from the body. Ultrafiltration is one of the two main functions of the *kidneys*. In *kidney failure*, problems with ultrafiltration result in *fluid overload*. *Dialysis* provides an alternative means of ultrafiltration.

Ultrasound scan A method of obtaining pictures of internal organs, such as the *kidneys*, or of an unborn baby, using sound waves. A device that sends out sound waves is held against the body. The sound waves produce echoes, which the scanner detects and builds up into pictures.

Under-dialysis Not having enough *dialysis*. If a dialysis patient does not achieve target blood levels for *creatinine*, the symptoms of *kidney failure* are likely to return. The amount of dialysis will then have to be increased.

Urea A substance made by the liver. It is one of the waste products from food that builds up in the blood when someone has kidney *failure*. Like *creatinine*, urea is a marker for other more harmful substances. The higher the urea level, the worse is the kidney failure.

Ureters The tubes that take *urine* from the *kidneys* to the *bladder*.

Urethra The body's tube that takes *urine* from the *bladder* to the outside of the body.

Urinary catheter A plastic tube inserted into the *bladder* for the removal of *urine*.

Urine The liquid produced by the *kidneys*, consisting of the toxic waste products of food and the excess water from the blood.

Vancomycin An *antibiotic drug*, commonly used to treat *peritonitis*, long-term *exit site* infections (of *peritoneal dialysis* catheters) and line (*haemodialysis catheter*) infections.

Vasodilator drugs Tablets that lower the *blood pressure* by making the *blood vessels* wider, so that the blood can flow through them more easily.

Veins *Blood vessels* which carry blood from the body back to the heart.

Virus A type of germ responsible for a range of mild and serious illnesses. Viruses are much smaller than *bacteria* and usually reproduce inside the cells of other living organisms.

Vitamin D A chemical that helps the body to absorb *calcium* from the diet. Blood levels of vitamin D are usually low in people with *kidney failure*.

Water tablets The common name for *diuretic drugs*.

White blood cells *Cells* in the blood that normally help to fight infection. They are part of the *immune system*. After a *kidney* transplant, they can be a 'bad thing', as they may attack (reject) the new kidney.

Xenotransplantation The transplanting of tissues or organs from one animal into a human or other type of animal.

FURTHER READING

Juliet Auer, *Living Well with Kidney Failure*. Class Publishing.

Stewart Cameron, *Kidney Disease: the facts*. Oxford Medical Publications.

Stewart Cameron, *History of the Treatment of Kidney Failure by Dialysis*. Oxford University Press.

Charles Fox and Ragnar Hanas, *Type 2 Diabetes*. Class Publishing.

Helena Jackson, Annie Cassidy and Gavin James, *Eating Well with Kidney Failure*. Class Publishing.

Kevin Kendrick and Simon Robinson, *Their Rights: advance directives and living wills explored*. Age Concern Books.

Norman Levinski, *Ethics and the Kidney*. Oxford University Press.

Jeremy Levy, Julie Morgan and Edwina Brown, *Oxford Handbook of Dialysis*. Oxford University Press.

Renal Registry, *Renal Registry Report 2005*. Available on www.renalreg.com. (Earlier reports also available from the same site.)

Toni Smith and Nicky Thomas, *Renal Nursing*. Balliere Tindall.

Peter Sonksen, Charles Fox and Sue Judd, *Diabetes: the 'at your fingertips' guide*. Class Publishing.

Andy Stein and Janet Wild, *Kidney Dialysis and Transplants: the 'at your fingertips' guide*. Class Publishing.

Julian Tudor Hart and Tom Fahey, *High Blood Pressure: the 'at your fingertips' guide*. Class Publishing.

Jacob van Noordwijk, *Dialysing for Life*. Kluwer Academic Publishers.

USEFUL ADDRESSES AND WEBSITES

Addresses correct at time of going to press, but please note that all are subject to change from time to time.

Action on Smoking and Health (ASH)
102 Clifton Street
London EC2A 4HW
Tel: 020 7739 5902
Fax: 020 7613 0531
Helpline: 0800 169 0169
Website: www.ash.org.uk
Information on how smoking affects medical conditions.

Age Concern England
Astral House
1268 London Road
London SW16 4ER
Tel: 020 8765 7200
Fax: 020 8765 7211
Helpline: 0800 009 966
Website: www.ageconcern.org.uk
Provides advice on a range of subjects for people over 50. Publishes books and fact sheets, and provides services via local branches.

British Association for Counselling
BACP House
35–37 Albert Street
Rugby
Warwickshire CV21 2SG
Tel: 08788 550 899
Website: www.counselling.co.uk
Send s.a.e. for information about counselling services in your area, and publications list.

British Kidney Patient Association
Bordon
Hampshire GU35 9JZ
Tel: 01420 472021/2
Fax: 01420 475831
Website: www.britishkidney-pa.co.uk
Provides information and advice to people with kidney illnesses throughout the UK. Grants available.

Cancerlink
Macmillan Cancer Relief
89 Albert Embankment
London SE1 7UQ
Tel: 020 7840 7840
Fax: 020 7840 7841
Helpline: 0808 808 0000
Website: www.cancerlink.org
Helps cancer patients, families and carers with practical and emotional support.

Carers' National Association
20-25 Glasshouse Yard
London EC1A 4JT
Tel: 020 7490 8818
Fax: 020 7490 8824
Helpline: 0808 808 7777
Website: www.carersonline.org.uk
Offers information and support to all people who have to care for others due to medical or other problems. Has national headquarters, as listed below.

Carers Northern Ireland
58 Howard Street
Belfast BT1 6PJ
Tel: 028 9043 9843
Fax: 028 9043 9299
Helpline: 0808 808 7777
Website: www.carersonline.org.uk

Carers Scotland
91 Mitchell Street
Glasgow G1 3LN
Tel: 0141 221 9141
Fax: 0141 221 9140
Helpline: 0808 808 7777
Website: www.carersonline.org.uk

Crossroads – Caring for Carers
10 Regent Place
Rugby
Warwicks CV21 2PN
Tel: 0845 450 0350
Fax: 0845 450 6550
Helpline: 0845 450 0350
Website: www.crossroads.org.uk
Provides a paid, trained person to offer respite care in the home.

CRUSE – Bereavement Care
126 Sheen Road
Richmond
Surrey TW9 1UR
Tel: 020 8939 9530
Fax: 020 8940 7638
Helpline: 0870 167 1677
Website:
www.crusebereavementcare.org.uk
Offers information and practical advice. Sells literature and has local branches that provide one-to-one counselling to people who have been bereaved. Runs training in bereavement counselling for professionals.

Department for Work and Pensions
Helpline: 0800 137 177
Government information service offering advice on benefits for people with disabilities, and their carers.

Department of Health
Richmond House
79 Whitehall
London SW1A 2NS
Tel: 020 7210 4850
Website: www.dh.gov.uk

Depression Alliance
35 Westminster Bridge Road
London SE1 7JB
Tel: 020 7633 9929
Fax: 020 7633 0559
Helpline: 0845 123 2320
Website: www.depressionalliance.org.uk
Offers support and understanding to anyone affected by depression, and relatives who want help. Has a network of self help groups, correspondence schemes and a range of literature. Send s.a.e. for information.

Diabetes UK
10 Parkway
London NW1 7AA
Tel: 020 7424 1000
Fax: 020 7424 1000
Helpline: 0845 120 29 60
Website: www.diabetes.org.uk
Provides advice and information for people with diabetes and their families; has local support groups.

Disability Wales/Anabledd Cymru
Bridge House
Caerphilly Business Park
Van Road
Caerphilly
Mid Glamorgan CF83 3GW
Tel: 029 2088 7325
Fax: 029 2088 8702
Website: www.disabilitywales.org

Disabled Living Foundation
380–384 Harrow Road
London W9 2HU
Tel: 020 7289 6111
Helpline: 0845 130 9177
Website: www.dlf.org.uk
Provides information on all kinds of equipment to help people cope with a disability.

DVLA (Drivers and Vehicles Licensing Authority
Drivers Medical Group
DVLA
Swansea SA99 1TU
Tel: 01792 772151
Helpline: 0870 6000301
Website: www.dvla.gov.uk
Government office providing advice for drivers with special needs.

Employment Opportunities for People with Disabilities
35 New Broad Street
London EC2M 1 SL
Tel: 020 7448 5420
Fax: 020 7374 4893
Website: www.opportunities.org.uk

Eurodial
www.eurodial.org
The international dialysis organisation dedicated to the care and mobility of dialysis patients in Europe.

Globaldialysis
www.globaldialysis.com
Gives details of holidays and travel information for dialysis patients.

Kidney Cancer UK
9 Foxall Road
Timberley
Altrincham
Cheshire WA15 6RW
Tel: 01889 585801
Website: kcuk.org
Information and support for people with kidney cancer and their carers. Chat room available via the website.

Kidney Patient Information Websites

www.kidneydirections.com
Information for kidney patients and suggestions for ways to plan treatment.

www.kidneypatientguide.org.uk
Information for patients with kidney failure, and those who care for them.

www.kidneywise.com
Advice and support for those affected by kidney failure.

Kidney Research UK
King's Chambers
Priestgate
Peterborough PE1 1FG
Tel: 0845 070 7601
Helpline: 0845 300 14 99
Email: info@ kidneyresearchuk.org
Website: www.kidneyresearchuk.org
Funds research into kidney disease, its causes and treatment. Works to raise awareness of kidney disease.

Medic-Alert Foundation
1 Bridge Wharf
156 Caledonian Road
London N1 9UU
Tel: 020 7833 3034
Fax: 020 7278 0647
Website: www.medicalert.org.uk
Offers selection of jewellery with internationally recognised medical symbol: 24 hour emergency phoneline.

MIND (National Association for Mental Health)
15–19 Broadway
Stratford
London E15 4BQ
Tel: 020 8519 2122
Helpline: 0845 766 0163
Website: www.mind.org.uk
Mental health organisation working for a better life for everyone experiencing mental distress. Has information and offers support via local branches.

National Institute for Health and Clinical Excellence (NICE)
MidCity Place
71 High Holborn
London WC1V 6NA
Tel 020 7067 5800
Website: www.nice.org.uk

National Kidney Federation
6 Stanley Street
Worksop
Notts S81 7HX
Tel: 01909 487 795
Fax: 01909 481 723
Helpline: 0845 601 02 09
Email: nkf@kidney.org.uk
Website: www.kidney.org.uk
Aims to promote, throughout the United Kingdom, the welfare of people suffering from kidney disease or renal failure, and those relatives and friends who care for them.

NHS Direct
England and Wales: 0845 4647
Website: www.nhsdirect.nhs.uk
Speak to a nurse for some common-sense advice about your health.

NHS 24
Scotland: 0845 424 24 24
Website: www.nhsdirect.nhs.uk
Speak to a nurse for some common-sense advice about your health.

**NHS Organ Donor
Information Service**
Helpline: 0845 6060 400
Website: www.uktransplant.org.uk/
ukt/how_to_become_a_donor
*Provides information about donating
organs and how patients can benefit
from organ donation.*

Outsiders Club
Sex and Disability Helpline
Tuppy Owens
BCM Box Lovely
London WC1N 3XX
Tel: 0707 499 3527 (11 am–7 pm)
Website: www.outsiders.org.uk
*A national self-help organisation that
helps with sexual problems.*

Patients Association
PO Box 935
Harrow
Middlesex HA1 3YJ
Tel: 020 8423 9111
Fax: 020 8423 9119
Helpline: 0845 608 44 55
Website: www.patients-association.com
Provides advice on patients' rights.

**RADAR (Royal Association
for Disability and Rehabilitation)**
12 City Forum
250 City Road
London EC1V 8AF
Tel: 020 7250 3222
Fax: 020 7250 0212
Website: www.radar.org.uk
*Campaigns to improve the rights and
care of people with a disability. Sells
special key to access locked public
toilets for the disabled.*

**Registered Nursing Homes
Association**
15 Highfield Road
Edgbaston
Birmingham B15 3DU
Tel: 0121 454 2511
Fax: 0121 454 9032
Website: www.rnha.co.uk
*Information about registered nursing
homes in your area that meet the
standards set by the Association.*

Relate
Herbert Gray College
Little Church Street
Rugby
Warwickshire CV21 3AP
Tel: 01788 573 241
Fax: 01788 535 007
Information line: 0845 456 1310
Helpline: 0845 130 4010
Website: www.relate.org.uk
*Formerly the Marriage Guidance
Council. Offers relationship
counselling via local branches, and
publishes information on health,
sexual, self-esteem, depression,
bereavement and remarriage issues.*

**Renal Registry
of the United Kingdom**
Southmead Hospital
Southmead Road
Bristol BS10 5NB
Tel: 0117 959 5665
Fax: 0117 959 5664
www.renalreg.com
*Collects, analyses and presents data
about the incidence, clinical
management and outcome of renal
disease.*

Sexual Dysfunction Association
Windmill Place Business Centre
2–4 Windmill Lane
Southall UB2 4NU
Helpline: 0870 774 35 71
Website: www.sda.uk.net
*Association providing help and advice
on sexual and relationship problems.*

Tourism for All
Hawkins Suite
Enham Place
Enham Alamein
Andover SP11 6JS
Tel: 0845 124 99 74
Fax: 0845 124 99 72
Helpline: 0845 124 99 71
Website: www.holidaycare.org.uk
*Information and advice about
holidays, travel or respite care for
older or disabled people, and their
carers.*

UK Transplant
Communications Directorate
Fox Den Road
Stoke Gifford
Bristol BS34 8RR
Tel: 0117 975 7575
Fax: 0117 975 7577
Website: www.uktransplant.org.uk

**United Kingdom Register
of Counsellors**
BACP House
35–37 Albert Street
Rugby
Warwickshire CV21 2SG
Tel: 0870 443 5232
Fax: 0870 443 5161
*Part of British Association of
Counselling and Psychotherapy
Regulatory body which provides
details of registered counsellors who
offer safe and accountable practice.*

**Unrelated Live Transplant
Regulatory Authority (ULTRA)**
Room 423
Wellington House
13–155 Waterloo Road
London SE1 8UG
Tel: 020 7972 4524
Fax: 020 7972 1830
Website:
www.advisorybodies.doh.gov.uk/ultra

Vitalise
12 City Forum
250 City Road
London EC1V 8AF
Tel: 0845 345 1972
Fax: 0845 345 1978
Website: vitalise.org.uk
*Formerly known as The Winged
Fellowship Trust, this organisation
provides holidays and respite care for
disabled people and their carers.*

INDEX

Page numbers followed by italic *g* refer to glossary items

A

A2 (AII) antagonists 9
abdomen 148*g*
  and peritoneal dialysis 55, 62
acceptance, after diagnosis 109
access, haemodialysis 68, 70–1, 148*g*
  difficult 69–70, 74
  problems with 74–5
ACE (angiotensin-converting enzyme)
    inhibitors 9, 27, 148*g*
acetate 43
acid 42, 148*g*
acid balance, blood test for 47
acidity level 104
activity prioritising 114
acute 148*g*
acute kidney failure 4
adequacy (tests) 49, 148*g*
Advanced Directive 129
advice, conflicting 111
age
  and blood pressure 26
  and coping with kidney failure 111,
    112
  of donor, and transplant suitability 88
  of patient, and transplant suitability
    77
AIDS 32, 80, 87
alanine transaminase (ALT)
  blood tests 45, 47
  normal and target blood levels 45, 47
albumin 148*g*
  blood tests 44, 47
  low blood level 102
  normal and target blood levels 44, 47

alfacalcidol 38, 43, 148*g*
ALG (anti-lymphocyte globulin) 97,
    148*g*
alkali 148*g*
alkaline phosphatase
  blood tests 45, 47
  normal and target blood levels 45, 47
alpha-blocker drugs 28, 148*g*
alprostadil 120
aluminium hydroxide 37, 148*g*
amino acids 12, 61, 148*g*
amlodipine 28
amyloid 38–9
anaemia 4, 30, 45, 148*g*
  erythropoietin treatment 24, 30,
    32–3
  key facts 34
  and poor appetite 30, 104
  after transplantation 33
  what it is 30–1
Andropatch 119
angina 119
angiogram 148*g*
  see also renal angiogram
angiotensin-converting enzyme (ACE)
    inhibitors 9, 27, 148*g*
angiotensin II (AII) antagonist 28, 148*g*
ankle oedema (swelling) 4, 5, 21, 74,
    148*g*
antibiotic drugs 75, 148*g*
  for exit site infections 64
  for peritonitis 64
  for tunnel infection 65
antibodies 32, 148*g*
  and cross-match 83
antigens 79, 148*g*
anti-lymphocyte globulin (ALG) 97,
    148*g*

anti-thymocyte globulin (ATG) 97, 148*g*
anxiety
  and blood pressure 26
  and kidney failure 110
APD (automated peritoneal dialysis) 53,
    59, 148*g*
  compared with CAPD 59–60
  portable APD machine 59
appetite, poor 5, 30, 104
Aranesp 32, 34
ARB *see* A2 (AII) antagonists
arteries 24, 148*g*
  and fistulas 68–9
  narrow 27
arteriovenous fistula (AVF) *see* fistulas
artificial kidney 148*g*
  see also dialyser (artificial kidney)
aspirin 100
atenolol 28, 117
ATG (anti-thymocyte globulin) 97, 148*g*
atheroma 6, 148*g*
atherosclerosis 6
automated peritoneal dialysis (APD) 58,
    59, 148*g*
  compared with CAPD 59–60
  portable APD machine 59
AVF (arteriovenous fistula) *see* fistulas
azathioprine 45, 98, 148*g*
  side effects 99

B

bacteria 149*g*
bags, dialysis *see* dialysis bags
basiliximab 98
baths, and peritoneal dialysis 61–2
bereavement 111
beta-blocker drugs 28, 149*g*
  causing erectile dysfunction 117

bicarbonate 149g
  blood tests 42–3, 47
  in dialysis fluid 61
  normal and target blood levels 42–3, 47
bilirubin
  blood tests 45, 47
  normal and target blood levels 45, 47
biochemistry blood tests 40, 41, 149g
biopsy 149g
  see also kidney (renal) biopsy
bisoprolol 28, 117
BK virus 100, 149g
bladder 1–2, 149g
bleeding, haemodialysis patients 75
blood
  circulation 24–5
  composition of 31
  toxin removal 2–3
blood cells 31, 149g
  see also platelets; red blood cells;
    white blood cells
blood group 149g
  matching for transplantation 79
blood health, blood test for 47
blood level(s) 149g
  normal 47
blood pressure (BP) 149g
  control by kidneys 4
  diastolic 25, 26, 150g
  factors affecting 26, 27
  high 9, 24, 27, 27–8
  key facts 29
  of kidney donor 87, 89
  low 22, 24, 28
  measuring 25–6, 26
  normal 26
  rapid changes in 73
  systolic 25, 26, 156g
  taking control of 28
blood pressure tablets
  causing erectile dysfunction 117
  delaying dialysis 9
  types of 27–8

blood tests 40
  alanine transaminase 45
  albumin 44, 47
  alkaline phosphatase 45, 47
  aspartate transaminase (AST) 47
  bicarbonate 42–3, 47
  bilirubin 45, 47
  calcium 43, 47
  cholesterol 46, 47
  creatinine 13, 14, 41–2, 47
  dialysable substances 41–4, 47
  in erectile dysfunction 118
  ferritin 46, 47
  the 'figures' 40
  gamma-glutamyltransferase 45, 47
  glucose 43–4, 47
  haemoglobin 31, 45, 47
  key facts 50
  liver function tests 45, 47
  non-dialysable substances 44–5, 47
  parathyroid hormone 46, 47
  phosphate 42, 47
  potassium 41, 47
  relevant body areas 47
  results, normal and target 47
  sodium 43, 47
  urea 13, 14, 42, 47
blood transfusions, and anaemia 32
blood vessels 149g
  see also arteries; veins
body image 110
  problems with 62, 73, 122
bone health 4, 105
  blood tests for 47
bone marrow 31, 149g
  drugs suppressing activity in 99
  location 30
bone pain
  and dialysis amyloidosis 38–9
  and renal bone disease 35
BP see blood pressure
brain death 81, 149g
brain health, blood test for 47
breath, shortness of 4, 5, 21, 30

bromocriptine 119
bruit 69
bumetanide 21
burnout, and peritoneal dialysis 62

C

cabergoline 119
cadaveric kidneys, sources 81
cadaveric transplants 78, 80–1, 149g
  Asian/Black shortage of 87
  compared with living donor
    transplants 86, 87, 90
  UK donors/transplants/patients 140
Calcichew 37, 42, 43, 77, 105
calcium 149g
  blood tests 43, 47
  and bone health 4
  in diet 105
  normal and target blood levels 35, 43, 47
  and parathyroidectomy 38
  and renal bone disease 35, 37
calcium acetate 37, 149g
calcium antagonists 28, 149g
calcium carbonate 149g
  after parathyroidectomy 38
  in renal bone disease 37
  tablets 37, 42, 43, 77, 105
cancer
  deaths from 134
  and donor transplant suitability 87
  and immuno-suppressant drugs 100–1, 130
  lymphoma 101
  skin 101
candesartan 28
Candida albicans 64, 149g
CAPD (continuous ambulatory
  peritoneal dialysis) 149g
  compared with APD 59–60
  fluid exchange 58, 59
captopril 27
cardiac catheter test 80
carvedilol 28

catheters 149*g*
  urinary 93, 156*g*
  see also haemodialysis catheters; PD
    catheters
cells 149–50*g*
central venous pressure (CVP) line 93
chest X-ray 80, 89
cholesterol 150*g*
  blood tests 46, 47
  and high blood pressure 27
  normal and target blood levels 46,
    47
  and renovascular disease 6
chronic 150*g*
chronic kidney failure 1, 4, 7
  NSF quality requirement 145
Cialis (tadalafil) 118, 119
ciclosporin 45, 98, 150*g*
  side effects 99
circulation problems, after transplant
  100
clearance 150*g*
  creatinine clearance tests 13, 16, 17,
    49, 150*g*
  haemodialysis patients 17
  how it is measured 12–13
  key facts 18
  patients not on dialysis 16–17
  PD patients 17
  toxic wastes 2
  types of test 13–14
  urea clearance tests 13, 16, 17
  why it is measured 12
CMV (cytomegalovirus) 150*g*
cold ischaemia time 86
coldness, feeling of 5
computed tomography (CT) scan 48,
  89, 150*g*
concentration, poor 5, 111–12
concordance, lack of 110
consent to tests 46
constipation, and peritoneal dialysis 63
continuous ambulatory peritoneal
  dialysis (CAPD) 149*g*

compared with APD 59–60
  fluid exchange 58, 59
contraception 125
coping with kidney failure
  and diagnosis 109
  factors affecting 112–13
  problems 109–12
  strategies 113–14
creatinine 5, 150*g*
  clearance tests 13, 16, 17, 49, 150*g*
  measurement of 13
  normal production 12–13
  patient weight and 15
creatinine blood tests/levels 13, 14,
    41–2, 47
  before dialysis 14
  during dialysis 15, 17
  level after kidney donation 91
  levels during pregnancy 122
  levels in kidney failure 8
  normal and target levels 13, 15,
    41–2, 47
  starting dialysis 14–15
  after a transplant 15–16
creatinine clearance tests 13, 16, 17,
    49, 150*g*
cross-match 83, 89, 150*g*
crush fractures 100
CT (computed tomography) scan 48,
    89, 150*g*
cultural factors, in coping with kidney
    failure 113
cysts *see* polycystic kidney disease
    (PCKD)
cytomegalovirus (CMV) 80, 100, 150*g*

D
daclizumab 98
darbepoetin alfa 32, 34
death 126
  awareness of 110
  key facts 131
  from kidney failure 127, 134–5
  progression towards 127

dehydration 21–2, 150*g*
  treatment 22
denial 109, 113
dependency 110–11
depression 111
desensitisation 88
developments in patient care 139–47
diabetes mellitus 6–7, 75, 150*g*
  blood glucose 43, 44
  and donor transplant suitability 87
  drugs causing 99
  and haemodialysis problems 75
diabetic nephropathy 6–7, 150*g*
diabetic retinopathy 75
diagnosis of kidney failure 5
  initial reaction to 109
dialysate *see* dialysis fluid(s)
dialyser (artificial kidney) 66, 67, 150*g*
  types of 67
dialysis 7–8, 150*g*
  alternatives for frail/elderly patients
    11
  cannot cure kidney failure 1, 10
  decision not to start 127–8
  delaying 9
  diffusion in 52–3
  fluid removal 53
  how it works 51
  informed choice 126, 128–9
  key facts 54
  NSF standard 145
  patient survival after 87
  restarting 16
  starting 9, 14–15
  survival rates 132
  trial of 128
  what it is 51
  withdrawal 129–30
  see also haemodialysis; peritoneal
    dialysis
dialysis amyloidosis 38–9
dialysis bags
  delivery and storage 62
  size and strength 44, 54, 60

dialysis catheters *see* haemodialysis catheters; PD catheters
dialysis fluid(s) (dialysate) 51, 150*g*
  cloudy 64
  role of 51–2
  special types of 61
dialysis fluid exchange
  in APD 58, 59
  in CAPD 58, 59
  training patients to carry out 57–8
dialysis (kidney) machine 66, 150*g*
  how it works 67
dialysis membrane 51, 52, 150*g*
diastolic blood pressure 25, 26, 150*g*
diet 102
  during dialysis 103
  healthy eating guidelines 102
  individual recommendations 106
  key facts 107
  minerals 105–6
  before starting dialysis 103
  taking control of 107
  after transplant 107
  vitamin supplements 106
diffusion 41, 56, 67, 150–1*g*
  process of 52
  waste removal by 51, 52–3
diltiazem 28
disease management 114
diuretic drugs 21, 27, 151*g*
dizziness
  and dehydration 22
  and low blood pressure 22, 27
DMSA scan 6, 49
donor(s) 151*g*
  choice of 88
  dead 81
  heart-beating 81
  living 81
  matching 79–80
  non-heart-beating (asystolic) 81
  shortage of Asian 82
  transplant suitability 87–8
  see also living donor transplants

donor kidney 151*g*
Doppler scan 97, 151*g*
double J stent 93, 94, 95
doxazosin 28
drainage problems in PD 63
drink *see* fluid intake
driving after transplant operation 94
drug abuse 87
drugs *see* alpha-blocker drugs; antibiotic drugs; beta-blocker drugs; diuretic drugs; immuno-suppressant drugs; steroids; vasodilator drugs; *and individual drug names*
DTPA scan 49
dying, end of life care, NSF quality requirement 145

E
ECG (electrocardiogram) 80, 89, 151*g*
ECHO (echocardiogram) 80, 151*g*
echocardiogram (ECHO) 80, 151*g*
ED *see* erectile dysfunction
education 142–3
eGFR *see* estimated glomerular filtration rate
electrocardiogram (ECG) 80, 89, 151*g*
enalapril 27
end-stage renal disease (ESRD) 1, 151*g*
end-stage renal failure (ESRF) 1, 151*g*
energy supplements 105
epileptic fits 33
EPO *see* erythropoietin
Eprex 34
ErecAid 119, 120
erectile dysfunction (impotence) 116
  causes 117
  investigations 118
  treatment 118–21
erection, normal 117
ERF *see* established renal failure
erythropoietin (EPO) 31–2, 45, 77, 151*g*
  and anaemia 24, 30, 31–2, 32–3
  and ferritin level 46

  for frail/elderly patients 11
  and high blood pressure 24
  key facts 34
  and menstruation 123
  poor response to 33
  side effects 33
  who needs? 32–3
ESRD (end-stage renal disease) 1, 151*g*
ESRF (end-stage renal failure) 1, 151*g*
established renal failure (ERF) 151*g*
  purpose of 10–11
  treatment 7–9
  unknown causes of 7
  what it is 4–5, 7
  see also kidney failure
estimated glomerular filtration rate (eGFR) 5, 14, 16–17, 17–18, 151*g*
  levels in kidney failure 8
  starting dialysis 15
exercise, with peritoneal dialysis 61, 62
exercise tolerance tests 80, 89
exit site 151*g*
  infection 64–5, 75
Expert Patient Programme 146

F
fat, in diet 102
fatigue, and peritoneal dialysis 62
felodipine 28
femoral line 70
ferritin 151*g*
  blood tests 46, 47
  and EPO treatment 33
  normal and target blood levels 46, 47
ferrous sulphate tablets 33
fertility, female 122–3
fever 75
fibrin, blocking PD catheter 63
'figures' 40
fistulas 68–9, 151*g*
  brachial 69
  limited life of 75
  operation to create 68

fistulas (*cont'd*)
  problems with 69, 74–5
  radial 69
fits 33
FK506 (tacrolimus) 45, 98, 151*g*,
  156*g*
  side effects 99
flesh, and body fluid 19
flucloxacillin 151*g*
fluid, body
  and flesh 19
  removal of excess, by kidneys
    (ultrafiltration) 2, 3
fluid balance
  blood test for 47
  control of 20
  key facts 23
  and sodium 20–1
  taking control of 22
  what it is 19
fluid intake
  for haemodialysis patients 74
  restrictions on 106
fluid overload 4, 20, 27, 151*g*
  and haemodialysis 74
  and peritoneal dialysis 62
  treatment 21
  what it is 21
focal and segmental glomerulosclerosis
  (FSGS) 78, 92
follicle-stimulating hormone (FSH) 118
food *see* diet
food hygiene 107
fractures 4, 35, 100
FSGS (focal and segmental
  glomerulosclerosis) 78, 92
FSH (follicle-stimulating hormone) 118
furosemide 21, 151*g*

G

gamma-glutamyltransferase (gammaGT)
  blood tests 45, 47
  normal and target blood levels 45, 47
ganciclovir 100

gentamicin 151*g*
GFR (glomerular filtration rate) 151*g*
glomerulonephritis (GN) 5, 78, 151*g*
  mesangiocapillary 78
  see also focal and segmental
    glomerulosclerosis
glomerulus 3, 151*g*
glucose (sugar) 151*g*
  blood tests 43–4, 47
  in dialysis fluid 53–4
  normal and target blood levels 43–4,
    47
glucose polymer, in Icodextrin 61
goal setting 114
Goodpasture's disease 78
grafts 71, 74–5, 151*g*
  limited life of 75
grief, after diagnosis 109
GTN spray 119
gum hypertrophy 99

H

haemodialysis 151–2*g*
  access *see* access, haemodialysis
  amount of 71–2
  and body size 68, 71, 73
  clearance measurement 17
  compared with peritoneal dialysis 54
  creatinine levels 15
  dialysis membrane in 52
  dose calculation 71–2
  exit site infection 75
  and fluid overload 74
  home haemodialysis 72–3, 142,
    152*g*
  in hospital 71–2
  how it is done 68
  how it works 66–7
  key facts 76
  lifestyle changes 73
  line infection 75
  patients' control of life with 76
  problems with 73–4, 75–6
  satellite 72

  semi-permanent 70
  single-needle 71
  what it does 66
  who can be treated 66
haemodialysis catheters 70, 152*g*
  blocked 75
  double-barrelled 68, 70
  infections 33
  limited life of 75
  lines, entry positions for 70
  problems with 75
  replaced 75
  single-barrelled 71
  temporary 70, 75–6
haemodialysis unit 152*g*
haemoglobin (Hb) 30, 152*g*
  blood tests 31, 45, 47
  normal and target blood levels 45,
    47
haemolytic uraemic syndrome 78
Hb *see* haemoglobin
healthy eating guidelines 102
heart
  and blood circulation 24–5
  and blood pressure 27
  location 2
heart attack, increased risk of 27, 100
heart-beating donor 152*g*
heart disease
  deaths from 134, 134–5
  after transplant operation 100
heart health, blood test for 47
Henoch-Schönlein purpura 78
heparin 63, 70, 75
hepatitis 32, 45, 80, 87, 89, 152*g*
hernias, and peritoneal dialysis 63–4
hip pain 99
HIV (human immunodeficiency virus)
  32, 80, 87, 89, 152*g*
home haemodialysis 72–3, 142, 152*g*
hormonal disturbances 117
hormone treatment, in erectile
  dysfunction 118, 119
hormones 152*g*

hospice care 127
human immunodeficiency virus (HIV) 32, 80, 87, 89, 152g
Human Organ Transplant Act 1989 90
hydralazine 28
hygiene, importance of 75, 107
hyperkalaemia (excess potassium) 74
hyperparathyroidism 152g

I

Icodextrin 61
IgA nephropathy 78
immune system 96, 152g
    suppression see immuno-suppressant drugs
immuno-suppressant drugs 96, 98, 152g
    cancer and 100–1, 130
    delaying dialysis 9
    and peritonitis 64
    side effects 99–100
impotence see erectile dysfunction
independence
    and haemodialysis 73
    and peritoneal dialysis 55, 61
infection
    deaths from 134
    exit site 64–5, 75
    and haemodialysis 75–6
    line 75
    peritonitis 64
    after transplant 100
    tunnel 65
information 142–3
information seeking 113
insulin 44
Intensive Care Units (ICUs) 140
intravenous drip 93–4
intravenous pyelogram (IVP) 6, 48, 152g
intravenous urogram (IVU) 48
irbesartan 28
iron 152g
    blood test see ferritin

deficiency 33
    tablets and injections 33, 46
irritability 30
isotope GFR (glomerular filtration rate) 49
itching 5, 36, 38
IVP (intravenous pyelogram) 6, 48, 152g
IVU (intravenous urogram) 48

J

jaundice 45
joints, problems with 99
jugular line 70

K

kidney(s) 1, 3, 152g
    artificial see dialyser (artificial kidney)
    functions see kidney functions
    location 1, 2
    'small' 7
    structure 3
kidney (renal) biopsy 7, 46–8, 152g
    nephritis and 5
    and rejection 97
kidney disease, chronic, NSF quality requirements 145
kidney donors 152g
    see also donor(s)
kidney failure 4, 152g
    acute 4
    causes 5–7
    causes of death 134–5
    chronic 1, 4, 7, 145
    death from 127
    diagnosis 5
    international comparisons 135, 136
    key facts 11
    number of UK patients with 1
    progression of 7, 8
    signs of 8
    stages of 8
    survival chances 132–4
    symptoms 5, 7, 8

treatment see treatments for kidney failure
    see also established renal failure
kidney functions
    blood pressure control 4
    excess water removal 2, 3–4
    keeping bones healthy 4
    red blood cell manufacture 4
    toxic waste removal 2–3, 12
    urine production 1–2
kidney machine 152g
    see also dialysis (kidney) machine
kidney transplants 153g
    benefits 77
    number of 139–42
    see also transplant(s); transplant kidney; transplant operation; transplantation
kidney units see renal units

L

labetalol 28
lactate 43
legs
    cramps 5
    restless 5
LFTs (liver function tests) 153g
life expectancy 133
lifestyle changes
    haemodialysis 73
    with peritoneal dialysis 61–2
line infection 75, 153g
lipids 153g
lisinopril 27
liver, urea production 12
liver function tests (LFTs) 45, 47, 153g
living donor transplants 85
    benefits 85–6
    choice of donor 88
    compared with cadaveric transplants 86, 87, 90
    key facts 92
    number of 141
    patient survival after 86

living donor transplants (*cont'd*)
    preparation for 90–1
    rejection risk 92
    removal of kidney 91
    risks 85
    risks to donor 91
    risks to recipient 92
    tests for donors 88–9
    tests for recipient 88
    who can donate 87–8
living related transplants (LRTs) 78, 153*g*
living unrelated transplants (LURTs) 78, 89–90, 153*g*
Living Will 129
losartan 28
LRTs (living related transplants) 78, 153*g*
lungs, location 2
lupus nephritis 78
LURTs (living unrelated transplants) 78, 89–90, 153*g*
luteinising hormone (LH) 118
lymphocytes 96, 153*g*
lymphoma 101

M
MAG-3 scan 6, 49
magnetic resonance imaging (MRI) scan 49, 153*g*
malnutrition 42, 44, 102, 104, 153*g*
markers 13, 153*g*
medical team, lack of co-operation with 109–10
mefruside 21
membrane 153*g*
membranous nephropathy 78
menstrual periods 122–3
mesangiocapillary glomerulonephritis 78
methyldopa 28
methylprednisolone 97, 153*g*
metolazone 21
metoprolol 28, 117

micturating cystourethrogram 48
minoxidil 28
mmol/l (millimoles per litre) 153*g*
molecule 153*g*
moxonidine 28
MRI (magnetic resonance imaging) scan 49, 153*g*
muscles, creatinine production 12–13
MUSE (Medicated Urethral System for Erection) 120
mycophenolate mofetil 98, 153*g*
    side effects 99

N
National Institute for Health and Clinical Excellence (NICE) 153*g*
National Service Framework (NSF) 143–6
Neorecormon 34
nephr- 153*g*
nephrectomy 153*g*
    laparoscopic 91
    open 91
nephritis 5, 9, 153*g*
nephrologist 153*g*
nephrology 153*g*
nephrons 3
neutropenia 99
NHS Plan 139
NICE (National Institute for Health and Clinical Excellence) 153*g*
nifedipine 28
non-compliance *see* concordance
non-heart-beating donor 153*g*
NSF (National Service Framework) 143–6
nuclear medicine scan 48–9, 97, 153*g*
nutritional status 102
    blood test for 47
    see also diet; malnutrition

O
obesity 103
obstructive nephropathy 7, 153*g*

treating 10
oedema 153*g*
    ankle oedema 4, 5, 21, 74, 148*g*
    pulmonary oedema 21, 74, 155*g*
    see also fluid overload
oestradiol 124
OKT3 (orthoclone K T-cell receptor 3) antibody 97, 153*g*
    side effects 97
omentectomy 57
organ 153*g*
orthoclone K T-cell receptor 3 (OKT3) antibody 97, 153*g*
    side effects 97
osmosis 54, 154*g*
osteodystrophy *see* renal bone disease
osteoporosis 100
oxygen, in the blood 24–5, 30

P
pain
    bone pain 35, 38–9
    in hips 99
    after transplant operation 91
pancreas 43
parathyroid glands 154*g*
    location of 36, 46
    overactive 36
parathyroid hormone (PTH) 154*g*
    blood tests 37, 46, 47
    location 36
    normal and target blood levels 46, 47
    overactive 36
    and renal bone disease 36, 37, 38, 46
parathyroidectomy 38, 154*g*
patient care
    developments in 139–47
    end of life care, NSF quality requirement 145
    key facts 147
patient-centred service, NSF standard 145

patients
  choice 142–3
  involvement 146–7
  social circumstances 143
PCKD (polycystic kidney disease) 5–6,
    154g
PD see peritoneal dialysis
PD catheters 154g
  blocked 63
  and body image 62
  displaced 63
  leaking 63
  operation to insert 57
  poor drainage 63
  position inside body 57
  protection in sport 61
  removal of 64, 94
penile implants 118, 121
penile injection therapy 118, 120
penile insertion (transurethral) therapy
    118, 120–1
perindopril 27
peritoneal cavity 56, 154g
  location 56
peritoneal dialysis (PD) 154g
  clearance measurement 17
  compared with haemodialysis 54
  creatinine level 15
  and diabetes 75
  exit site infection 64–5
  how it is done 56–7
  how it works 55–6
  key facts 65
  lifestyle changes 61–2
  patient and family commitment 55
  problems with 62–3
  training in use of 57–8
  tunnel infection 65
  what it does 55
  who is suitable for 55
peritoneal dialysis catheters see PD
    catheters
peritoneal equilibration test (PET) 49,
    60, 154g

peritoneal function test (PFT) 49
peritoneum 52, 56, 154g
  how it works 60
  'wearing out' 63
peritonitis 33, 64, 154g
  affecting patient's suitability for
    transplant 64
personality, in coping with kidney failure
    112–13
PET (peritoneal equilibration test) 49,
    60, 154g
PFT (peritoneal function test) 49
phosphate 154g
  blood tests 42, 47
  and bone health 4
  in diet 105
  normal and target blood levels 36,
    42, 47
  and renal bone disease 35, 36, 37–8
phosphate binders 37, 105, 154g
plasma 4, 31, 154g
platelets 31, 99, 154g
polycystic kidney disease (PCKD) 5–6,
    154g
'postcode lottery' 136–7, 143
potassium 154g
  blood tests 41, 47
  in the diet 105–6
  excess (hyperkalaemia) 74
  normal and target blood levels 41, 47
prazosin 28
prednisolone 97, 98, 154g
  delaying dialysis 9
  side effects 98–9
pregnancy 123–5
preparation and choice, NSF standard
    145
prolactin 118, 119
propranolol 28, 117
prostate gland 7
protein(s) 154g
  and creatinine 13
  dietary 103, 104
  supplements 105

and urea 12, 14
  in urine 9, 91
proteinuria 9, 91
psychological aspects of kidney failure
    108
  diagnosis, initial reaction to 109
  key facts 115
  longer-term problems 109–12
  sexual problems 117, 122
  stresses 108–9
psychological assessments of
    donor/recipient 89
PTH see parathyroid hormone
pulmonary oedema 21, 74, 155g
pyelonephritis 6, 155g

Q
quality of life 126

R
radio-isotope scan 155g
radio-nuclide scan 155g
ramipril 27
recipient 155g
red blood cells 31, 155g
  lack of see anaemia
  role of 4, 30
  see also haemoglobin
reflux 6, 155g
reflux nephropathy 6, 155g
rejection, of transplant 96, 155g
  acute 96–7
  chronic 97–8
religious factors
  in coping with kidney failure 113
  in withdrawing from treatment 130–1
renal 155g
renal angiogram 6, 48, 89
renal biopsy see kidney (renal) biopsy
renal bone disease (osteodystrophy) 4,
    155g
  causes 35–6
  development of 35
  and EPO treatment 33

renal bone disease (*cont'd*)
key facts 39
monitoring 37
and parathyroid hormone (PTH) 36, 37, 38, 46
and transplants 38
treatment 37–8
renal failure *see* established renal failure; kidney failure
Renal National Service Framework (NSF) 143–6
renal networks 144
renal services 146
international comparisons 136
renal units 139, 155*g*
renovascular disease 6, 155*g*
residual renal function (RRF) 49, 155*g*
resources, availability of 142
rifampicin 155*g*
rigors 75, 155*g*
RRF (residual renal function) 49, 155*g*

S
salt
and blood pressure 28
reducing intake 20–1, 21, 27, 43, 102, 106
see also sodium
satellite haemodialysis unit 72, 155*g*
scan 155*g*
scrotal leak 63
self-confidence, loss of 110–11
semi-permeable 155*g*
sevelamer 37
sexual activity 111
with peritoneal dialysis 62
after transplant operation 94
sexual problems 116
emotional problems 121
investigating 116
key facts 125
sex drive, loss/reduction of 5, 30, 111, 121–2
in women 121–2

see also erectile dysfunction
shivering 75
shock, after diagnosis 109
showers, and peritoneal dialysis 61–2
sidofovir 100
sildenafil (Viagra) 118, 119
sirolimus 98, 155*g*
side effects 99
skin, pale 30
skin cancer 101
sleeping, poor 5
smoking 6, 27, 100
social factors, in coping with kidney failure 113
sodium 155*g*
blood tests 43, 47
normal and target blood levels 43, 47
see also salt
sodium profiling 74
sphygmomanometer 25–6, 155*g*
spiritual concerns
in coping with kidney failure 113
in withdrawing from treatment 130–1
sport, and peritoneal dialysis 61
Staphylococcus 64, 155*g*
statins 46, 100, 156*g*
statistics 132–8
key facts 138
steal syndrome 69
stem cells 82
steroids 97, 98
side effects 100
stress, on kidney patients 108–9
stroke
deaths from 134
increased risk of 27, 100
subclavian line 70
sugar *see* glucose
sugar diabetes *see* diabetes mellitus
support
in coping with kidney failure 113
in renal units 72
survival chances 132–4
sweating 20

swimming, and peritoneal dialysis 61–2
symptoms of kidney failure 5, 7, 8
systolic blood pressure 25, 26, 156*g*

T
tablets *see* drugs
tacrolimus (FK506) 45, 98, 151*g*, 156*g*
side effects 99
tadalafil (Cialis) 118, 119
telmisartan 28
terazosin 28
testosterone 117, 118, 119
thinking positively 114
thrombocytopenia 99
tiredness 5
anaemia and 4, 30
and EPO treatment 32
and erectile dysfunction 117
tissue 156*g*
tissue matching 89
tissue type 156*g*
matching 79–80
tissue typing 89, 156*g*
toxins 156*g*
blood tests for 47
build-up of 2–3, 12
in kidney failure 2–3
removal of *see* clearance
transplant(s) 156*g*
cadaveric 149*g*
international comparisons 137–8
living donor or cadaveric? 90
withdrawal from treatment after 130
see also kidney transplants; living donor transplants; living related transplants; living unrelated transplants
transplant kidney 156*g*
buying, selling and donating 90
how long it lasts 86, 94–6
position in body 95
sources 80–2
transplant operation 83, 93, 95, 156*g*
benefits of 77

transplant operation (*cont'd*)
  cancer after 100–1
  creatinine levels after 15–16
  dialysis before 78–9
  driving after 94
  heart disease after 100
  infection after 100
  key facts 101
  monitoring after 94
  pain after 91
  post-operative tubes 93–4
  problems after 96–101
  rejection 96–8
  and renal bone disease 38
  sex after 94
  tests before 83
  who can have 77
transplant waiting list 78, 82, 156*g*
transplantation 9, 156*g*
  effect on anaemia 33
  finding a suitable kidney 79–80
  key facts 84
  matching the blood group 79
  matching the tissue type 79–80
  not a cure for kidney failure 1, 10
  NSF standard 145
  suitability tests 80
  testing for viruses 80
transporters, high/low 60
treatment
  changes to 111
  stopped, death after 134
treatments for kidney failure
  cannot cure 1, 10
  reasons for 10–11
  stages 8
  see also dialysis; haemodialysis;
    peritoneal dialysis; transplant
    kidney; transplant operation;
    transplantation
tunnel infection 65, 156*g*

U
UKT (United Kingdom Transplant)
  156*g*
ULTRA (Unrelated Living Transplant
  Regulatory Authority) 90, 156*g*
ultrafiltration 67, 156*g*
  fluid removal by 53–4
  in healthy kidneys 2, 3
  process of 53
ultrasound scan 49, 156*g*
  and kidney donation 89
  and pyelonephritis 6
  after transplantation 97
under-dialysis 33, 156*g*
unit haemodialysis 72
United Kingdom Transplant (UKT)
  156*g*
Unrelated Living Transplant Regulatory
  Authority (ULTRA) 90, 156*g*
urea 12, 103, 156*g*
  blood tests 13, 14, 42, 47
  clearance tests 13, 16, 17
  during dialysis 17
  measurement of 13
  normal level 13
  normal and target blood levels 42, 47
urea kinetic modelling 16, 71–2
urea reduction ratio (URR) 71
ureters 1, 2, 156*g*
urethra 1, 2, 156*g*
urinary catheters 93, 156*g*
urinary system 1–2
  location 2
urine 156–7*g*
  functions 2
  production, normal 1–2
  protein in 9

V
vacuum devices, in erectile dysfunction
  118, 119–20
vancomycin 64, 157*g*
vasodilator drugs 157*g*
  types 27–8

veins 25, 157*g*
  and fistulas 68–9
Viagra (sildenafil) 118, 119
virus 157*g*
viruses, tests before transplantation 80
vitamin D 157*g*
  after parathyroidectomy 38
  and renal bone disease 35, 36, 37,
    38
  tablets 43
  see also alfacalcidol
vitamin supplements 106

W
waste removal
  by healthy kidneys 2–3
  see also clearance
water, excess *see* fluid, body
water loss 20
water tablets 157*g*
  see also diuretic drugs
weakness 5
  and dehydration 22
  and low blood pressure 22, 27
weight
  and amount of body fluid 19
  and amount of haemodialysis 71
  gain 103
  haemodialysis and body size 68, 71,
    73
  and high blood pressure 27
  loss 103, 104–5
  'target' (dry/ideal) 20
  and target creatinine 15
white blood cells 31, 157*g*

X
X-rays 48
  cardiac catheter test 80
  chest 80, 89
xenotransplantation 81–2, 157*g*

The *Class Health* Feedback Form

We hope that you found this *Class Health* book helpful. We always appreciate readers' opinions and would be grateful if you could take a few minutes to complete this form for us.

❶ How did you acquire your copy of this book?

From my local library ☐

Read an article in a newspaper/magazine ☐

Found it by chance ☐

Recommended by a friend ☐

Recommended by a patient organisation/charity ☐

Recommended by a doctor/nurse/adviser ☐

Saw an advertisement ☐

❷ How much of the book have you read?

All of it ☐

More than half of it ☐

Less than half of it ☐

❸ Which copies/chapters have been most helpful?

....

....

....

❹ Overall, how useful to you was this *Class Health* book?

Extremely useful ☐

Very useful ☐

Useful ☐

❺ What did you find most helpful?

....

....

....

❻ What did you find least helpful?

....

....

....

❼ What did you find least helpful?

....

....

....

❽ Have you read any other health books?

Yes ☐   No ☐

If yes, which subjects did they cover?

....

....

How did this *Class Health* book compare?

Much better ☐

Better ☐

About the same ☐

Not as good ☐

❾ Would you recommend this book to a friend?

Yes ☐   No ☐

Thank you for your help. Please send your completed form to:

Class Publishing, FREEPOST, London W6 7BR

Surname   First name

Title: Prof/Dr/Mr/Mrs/Ms

Address

Town   Postcode

Country

☐ Please add my name and address to receive details of related books

[Please note, we will not pass on your details to any other company]

Have you found **Kidney Failure Explained** useful and practical? If so, you may be interested in other books from Class Publishing.

Eating Well with Kidney Failure

Helena Jackson, Annie Cassidy and Gavin James £14.99

If you have kidney failure, you need to adapt and change what you eat. But, as this practical and exciting new book shows, you don't need to go on a crash diet, or to deny yourself the foods you love – you just need to adapt your favourite recipes with kidney-friendly foods. You can eat well, enjoy your food, and give your body the nutrition it needs.

This brilliant book provides a clear and practical guide to eating well with kidney failure, as well as a collection of more than fifty delicious recipes to show you how it all works in practice. The recipes have been analysed for their nutritional content and are coded to help you choose the most appropriate dishes for your individual requirements.

Living Well with Kidney Failure

Juliet Auer £14.99

This practical and inspiring book will give you the confidence to live a full and rewarding life. It highlights the experiences of a number of very different people, from all walks of life, ages and family situations. These shared personal accounts celebrate the fullness of life that people living with kidney failure can, and do, achieve.

'This cheerful book will be a great help and encouragement to patients and their families trying to become experts on renal failure.'
Dr Christopher Winearls,
Clinical Director of the Oxford Kidney Unit

Kidney Dialysis and Transplants – the 'at your fingertips' guide

Dr Andy Stein and Janet Wild with Juliet Auer £14.99

A practical handbook for anyone with long-term kidney failure or their families. The book contains answers to over 450 real questions actually asked by people with end-stage renal failure, and offers positive, clear and medically accurate advice on every aspect of living with the condition.

'A first class book on kidney dialysis and transplants that is simple and accurate, and can be used to equal advantage by doctors and their patients.'
Dr Thomas Stuttaford,
The Times

Diabetes – the 'at your fingertips' guide

Professor Peter Sonksen, Sue Judd and Dr Charles Fox £14.99

This is an invaluable reference guide for people with diabetes. It offers practical advice on every aspect of living with the condition, giving you the knowledge and reassurance you need to deal confidently with your diabetes.

'I have no hesitation in commending this book.'
Sir Steve Redgrave CBE,
Vice President, Diabetes UK

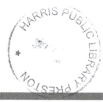

PRIORITY ORDER FORM

Cut out or photocopy this form and send it (*post free in the UK*) to:

Class Publishing Priority Service
FREEPOST 16705
Macmillan Distribution
Basingstoke, RG21 6ZZ

Tel: 01256 302 699
Fax: 01256 812 558

Please send me urgently
(*tick below*)

Post included price
per copy (UK only)

☐ **Kidney Failure Explained**
(ISBN 10: 1859591450 / ISBN 13: 9781859591451)   £20.99

☐ **Eating Well with Kidney Failure**
(ISBN 10: 1859591167 / ISBN 13: 9781859591161)   £17.99

☐ **Living Well with Kidney Failure**
(ISBN 10: 1859591124 / ISBN 13: 9781859591123)   £17.99

☐ **Kidney Dialysis and Transplants – the 'at your fingertips' guide**
(ISBN 10: 1859590462 / ISBN 13: 9781859590461)   £17.99

☐ **Diabetes – the 'at your fingertips' guide**
(ISBN 10: 185959087X / ISBN 13: 9781859590874)   £17.99

TOTAL _____

Easy ways to pay

Cheque: I enclose a cheque payable to Class Publishing for £ _____

Credit card: please debit my   ☐ Mastercard   ☐ Visa   ☐ Amex

Number _____   Expiry date _____

Name _____

My address for delivery is _____

_____

Town _____   County _____   Postcode _____

Telephone number (in case of query) _____

Credit card billing address if different from above _____

Class Publishing's guarantee: remember that if, for any reason, you are not satisfied with these books,
we will refund all your money, without any questions asked. Prices and VAT rates may be altered for
reasons beyond our control.